The New Truth
About Vitamins & Minerals

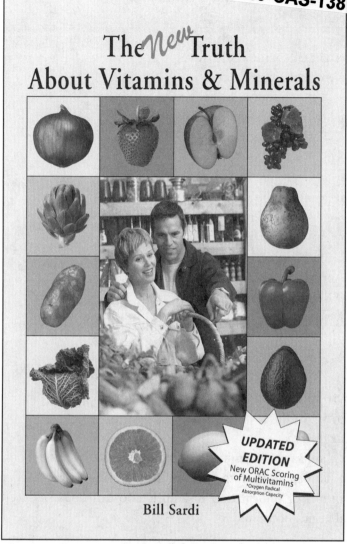

UPDATED
EDITION
New ORAC Scoring
of Multivitamins
*Oxygen Radical
Absorption Capacity

Bill Sardi

*Americans aren't eating fruits and vegetables,
so now they are being urged to take multivitamins,
but are they taking the right ones?*

Includes Survey of Top Brands of Multivitamins

by Bill Sardi

The New Truth About Vitamins & Minerals
by Bill Sardi

© Copyright Bill Sardi 2003
    www.askbillsardi.com

Published by Here & Now Books
        457 West Allen Avenue #117
        San Dimas, CA 91773

Cover designer and book layout:
        Sand Dollar Marketing, www.sdmllc.com

First Edition Printing:
        April 2003
Second Edition Printing:
        May 2004

A.D.A.M. Images © Copyright 2003 A.D.A.M., Inc.

Other Titles from Bill Sardi:
The Bible Prescription for Health and Longevity
The Power of Healing, The Power of God
How to Live 100 Years Without Growing Old
The Iron Time Bomb
In Search of the World's Best Water
Why Babies Die
The Anti-Aging Pill

Table of Contents

Introduction

A remarkable change is underway. In sedentary, well-nourished populations in developed countries, poor food choices abound and obesity rates are rising. Advice to eat fresh fruits and vegetables is being ignored. French fries have become the most common vegetable consumed in America. A recent survey showed that 77 percent of people who eat French fries would continue to do so even if they found they caused cancer. Human beings are falling victim to abundance and their own taste buds. Refined sugars, saturated and hydrogenated fats, iron, salt and calcium predominate over antioxidants and B vitamins. The result is humankind is regressing rather than advancing from a nutritional standpoint. Humans are devolving, not evolving. People living in undeveloped lands who eat more raw plant foods have far lower rates of disease than in developed countries.

> *In spite of nutritional breakthroughs, multivitamins remain unchanged*

Health authorities, resigned to admit their efforts to encourage Americans to eat more fresh fruits and vegetables have failed, have now come to realize human populations are going to have to rely upon vitamin pills to make up for nutritional shortages in their diets. After decades of telling the public all they needed was a good diet to meet their nutritional needs, the American Medical Association has done an about face and recommended multivitamins. But are Americans taking the right vitamins and minerals? The answer is no.

In spite of nutritional breakthroughs, particularly those involving folic acid, vitamin D and vitamin C, and a greater understanding of the science behind vitamin E, vitamin A and various minerals, for the most part brands of multivitamins remain largely unchanged. Few if any companies modify their products based upon revelations from the scientific literature. Remarkably few companies have even heeded the

< 5 >

advice provided freely in my first survey of multivitamins (WHAT'S BEST IN MULTIVITAMINS).

If consumers were confused about vitamin supplements in the past, they should be more confused today. There is considerable disagreement between authorities over

Doctors mention multivitamins less than one percent of the time

whether the public should take multivitamins or not. While the American Medical Association (AMA) has done an about face and now recommends multivitamins for every American [J Am Med Assn 287: 3116-26, 2002], the National Academy of Sciences continues to say that daily nutrient requirements can be met, in almost all instances, without taking supplements. Who's advice do we follow? Furthermore, despite reams of evidence to the contrary, the AMA says health-conscious consumers only need take low-dose, dime-a-day multivitamins and that so-called *"mega-vitamin"* supplements are a waste of money.

How are consumers to understand the lingo that surrounds vitamin labels, the Recommended Daily Allowance (RDA), the new Reference Daily Intake (RDI), the newly published Tolerable Upper Limits (UL), and compare them with Daily Values used for portions of foods?

When consumers read labels on multivitamin bottles and they indicate a particular nutrient is provided in a dosage that meets 100 percent of the Recommended Daily Allowance, should they believe that amount is enough to maintain optimal health? If more than the RDA is provided, should consumers conclude that the product provides excessive dosage and they are paying for vitamins they don't need? But the Recommended Dietary Allowance reflects the levels of intake of essential nutrients *"judged by the Food & Nutrition Board to be adequate to meet the known nutrient needs of practically all healthy persons."* The catch is the word *"healthy."*

< 6 >

How many Americans are perfectly healthy?

How many Americans are perfectly healthy? Out of a population of 280 million people, 50 million have heart disease, 43 million have high blood pressure, 15.7 million are diabetic, 33 million are hospitalized annually, 4 million are pregnant or lactating females, 66 million smoke tobacco, 34 million are of advanced age and have extra need for nutrients. Add to these numbers many millions of

There are organized efforts to restrict the dosage of vitamins

adults who take medications that deplete the body of essential nutrients. Fewer than one in five Americans consumes the five servings of fresh fruits and vegetables recommended by health authorities. This very fact is what prompted the American Medical Association to change its mind regarding vitamin and mineral supplementation. The medical profession now has to play catch up. Despite the widespread need, <u>out of some 823 million visits to office-based doctors in the year 2000, multivitamins were only mentioned in 1.5 percent of the time.</u> [Advance Data No. 328, June 5, 2002] Physicians continue to prescribe drugs that are fraught with potential side effects while advising their patients to be wary of vitamin tablets. Even more disheartening is the fact that many patients know more than their doctors about nutrition.

Tolerable Upper Limit

In the near future consumers may observe that vitamin and mineral supplements labels include a new piece of information, something called Tolerable Upper Limits. The inclusion of upper dosage limits on multivitamins is likely to be mistakenly construed by consumers as the point where toxicity begins. Actually, the Tolerable Upper Limit established by the Institutes of Medicine is intended to ensure that supplement users will not experience adverse effects. There is a cushioning or safety factor of 1 to 5 before real adverse symptoms occur. The Tolerable Upper Intake Level is the *"maximum level of daily nutrient intake that is unlikely to pose risks of adverse health effects to almost all of*

< 7 >

the individuals in the group for whom it is designed." [Food & Nutrition Board, Natl Acad Sci] <u>The Tolerable Upper Limit is actually the Tolerable Safe Upper Limit which does not even approach toxicity</u>. But consumers are likely to be misled by this labelling. News reports citing the Tolerable Upper Limits mistakenly warn consumers away from what is entirely safe. Furthermore, Tolerable Upper Limits do not disclose the severity of any potential adverse effect. Most side effects produced by vitamins and minerals are transient like diarrhea, finger tingling, or skin flushing and even in the case of liver toxicity are reversible. The Tolerable Upper Limit is likely to incorrectly scare patients away from vitamin supplements.

By increasing the daily dose of vitamins and minerals in supplements, therapeutic benefits may often be realized. <u>The establishment of upper limits on vitamin and mineral supplements comes at a time when scientific studies are revealing more health benefits when supplements are taken in safe mega-doses</u>. For example, 500 mg of vitamin C and 300 mg of vitamin B6 may reduce blood pressure, particularly among adults who have high sugar levels, and avert the need for costly and problematic prescription drugs. [Am J Therapy 9: 289-93, 2002; Mol Cell Biochem 200: 155-62, 1999]

A more disturbing problem is that of a worldwide effort to *"harmonize"* the dosage of vitamin and mineral supplements to levels that would only prevent deficiency diseases such as scurvy, pellagra, rickets and beri beri. Nutritional requirements vary from country to country. For example, vitamin A is desperately needed in undeveloped lands, but in the US, dietary consumption levels of vitamin A exceed the Recommended Daily Allowance. The needed amount of iron in developing countries is not the same in developed countries. Where the lifespan is longer there is the danger of iron overload. In northern climates where there is cloud cover for much of the year there is a greater need for vitamin D, much more so than among human populations near the Equator where intense UV rays produce more vitamin D via the skin. Harmonization of vitamin and mineral dosages will not universally meet the nutritional needs of all people.

< 8 >

Furthermore, trade agreements (CODEX) would relinquish the establishment of dosage limits for US-made vitamin supplements to foreign dictocrats at the United Nations and the World Health Organization. Vitamin supplements would be in control of foreigners who are not subject to any oversight by elected officials.

Restricted dosage

An example of the effort to confine vitamin supplements to very low doses burst into view when the British Foods Standards Agency attempted to restrict the dosage of B6 to no more than 10 milligrams in food supplements. [Warning on Vitamin Use, BBC News, August 30, 2002] A group of 220 doctors widely objected to the proposed 10 milligram limit for B6 and wrote a memorandum

Food supplements are far safer than foods

to the British House of Commons Agriculture Select Committee in June of 1998. [The Lancet, Volume 351, No. 9115, May 1998] However, some authorities suggest the public is misled over health benefits from vitamin B6 and that labels on bottles of vitamin B6 should include the caveat *"of unproven usefulness."*

The proposed restriction on vitamin B6 defies scientific understanding. The US National Academy of Sciences concluded that there was no convincing evidence of adverse reactions in doses up to 200 milligrams per day. Then a margin for safety was calculated at half that dose and the 100 milligram suggested maximum daily intake was established in the US. The Expert Group on Vitamins and Minerals in Great Britain issued a paper citing in detail various studies involving vitamin B6 toxicity which confirms reversible nerve toxicity (finger tingling) really doesn't begin till 200 milligrams are consumed for a prolonged period of time. [EVM/00/19, Revised August 2002]

There must be some other reason why authorities would limit the dosage of vitamin B6. It turns out that vitamin B6 when taken in safe mega-doses could quell many millions of cases of high blood pressure.

< 9 >

High blood sugar levels increase levels of aldehyde which raises blood pressure. Vitamin B6 lowers aldehyde levels. When small animals prone to develop high blood pressure were given 20 times the recommended dietary intake of vitamin B6 they did not develop hypertension. The conclusion of this study was that supplemental vitamin B6 *"may be an effective anti-hypertensive."* [Molecular Cell Biochemistry, Volume 200, pages 155-62, October 1999] This would be equivalent to about 34 to 40 milligrams of vitamin B6 in humans. In another animal study, obese rodents supplied with five times the normal intake of vitamin B6 experienced complete resolution of hypertension in 3-4 weeks. The removal of vitamin B6 resulted in the return of hypertension within two weeks. [Journal Hypertension, Volume 14, pages 355-63, March 1996] In a human study, 5 milligrams of vitamin B6 per kilogram of body weight (2.2 lbs) was administered orally for four weeks which resulted in a significant reduction in blood pressure. In this study, a 160-pound individual would have received 363 milligrams of vitamin B6. [Arzneimittelforschung, Volume 45, 1271-73, 1995] That much vitamin B6 may not be needed by the average hypertensive patient since most cases involve marginally elevated blood pressure.

If vitamin B6 tablets are only made available in 10 mg tablets, or even 25 mg tablets, this means a person with high blood pressure might have to take 12-40 B6 pills a day which would be as costly as blood pressure drugs and more inconvenient. Blood pressure medications are likely to cost consumers over $1000 a year whereas vitamin B6 pills would cost less than $100 a year.

Recall that the reason health authorities want to limit vitamin B6 is to avoid finger tingling. Compare this reversible minor side effect with those of medications used to control high blood pressure. ACE inhibitors, which are the most commonly prescribed drug for this condition, may accelerate kidney failure and may cause a profound drop in blood pressure among diabetics who also take water pills (diuretics). Diuretics are considered first-line treatment of hypertension, but the dose of diuretics must be kept low so as not to cause loss of potassium, sodium and magnesium which could induce irregular heart

< 10 >

rhythm. Beta blocking drugs are also employed but there is concern over their usefulness and they may reduce blood flow in peripheral blood vessels. It is obvious the side effects of commonly-used blood pressure lowering drugs are far greater in severity and frequency than the *"finger tingling"* that occurs with use of high-dose vitamin B6.

Vitamins held to a higher standard: absolute safety

Another problem is that the medical profession appears to hold vitamin and mineral supplements to a higher standard than prescription medications. There is no substance, including water, which is absolutely safe. Drugs, vitamins, even foods, are only relatively safe. For comparison, food supplements are far safer than foods. There are over 76 million cases of food poisoning annually in the US which causes 5000 deaths. [Centers for Disease Control] Yet consumers may hear exaggerated reports of potential liver toxicity from high-doses of vitamin A. Yet no person has ever died taking vitamin A tablets and the 50-60 cases of liver toxicity associated with vitamin A supplements reported annually in the USA occur largely among adults with pre-existing liver disease or misguided individuals who mistakenly overdose. The side effects of vitamin A overdose are completely reversible and are not lethal.

For comparison, the Poison Control Centers of America report on the number of reported problems and deaths in 2001 from the following substances:

< 11 >

	Number of adverse reports	Number of deaths
Multivitamins	2811	0
Oral contraceptives	9948	1
Insulin	1686	8
Diuretics (water pills)	7710	10
Cough and cold preparations	97710	14
Aspirin (adult)	5249	14
Acetaminophen (Tylenol)	28991	63
Alcohol	40782	93
Antidepressants	92675	255
Source: Am J Emerg Med 20: 391-452, 2002		

If a patient arrives at a doctor's office with a side effect from taking vitamins, it may be published as a case report in a medical journal. Front-page news stories may even be generated over one or two reported side effects alleged to be related to vitamin supplements. Yet, on a relative basis, even over-the-counter medications are far more risky than multivitamins. Even properly-prescribed prescription drugs, administered by nurses in hospitals, are responsible for over 100,000 mortal events a year (that's 274 needless fatalities a day!). [J Am Med Assn 279: 1200-05, 1998]

> **Consumers have won the right to have bonafide health claims printed on labels**

More regulation or less?

The frequently-heard argument is that vitamin pills are unregulated and that the Food & Drug Administration needs to step in and invoke greater regulatory measures over food supplements. The regulated-drug industry is not worth modeling food supplements after. Over $177 billion of side effects are generated from $100 billion of annual sales of

< 12 >

prescription drugs. [J Am Pharma Assn 40: 192, 2001] Often the side effects are worse than the remedy.

This is not to say that quality assurance of food supplements does not stand in need of improvement. It simply means <u>more regulation will likely raise prices and result in little increased safety given the extremely low rate of serious side effects with multivitamins</u>. One of the false allegations against food supplements is that they are not proven to be effective. First, to name just a few nutrients, there is ample data extolling the effectiveness of vitamin C, folic acid, magnesium, vitamin B6 and selenium, even in high doses. Second, why aren't more research dollars directed toward the study of food supplements so effectiveness can be further confirmed? Third, the pharmaceutical model of proving effectiveness requires millions of dollars which would make vitamins and minerals prescription drugs! From time to time there are recalls of prescription drugs because of manufacturing problems, but there is no call for greater regulation of the pharmaceutical industry. For example, the manufacturer of synthetic thyroid hormone (Synthroid) was challenged because its formula had changed numerous times and many manufacturing lots were recalled due to subpotent doses. Drug regulators said Synthroid was *"not reliably potent or stable."* This hormone was permitted to be marketed at sub-effective doses even when alternatives existed. Would a food supplement be given the same latitude? There appears to be two standards, one for drugs and another for food supplements. Furthermore, if food supplement manufacturers produce products that even produce innocuous side effects, consumers are unlikely to keep using them. The marketplace would eliminate inferior products.

News reporters continually cite data that 2500 adverse events resulting in 79 deaths occurred from the use of dietary supplements. Over 900 of these adverse reports and 44 deaths involved people taking just one herbal product, ephedrine-like stimulants commonly used for weight loss, and most of these cases are believed to have involved intentional mis-use (exceeding recommended daily dosage). [Associated Press, Feb.

< 13 >

22, 1998] For comparison, ephedrine or synthetic ephedrine is found in cold preparations and decongestants and causes no alarm.

Regarding the adverse events and alleged fatalities mentioned above, these figures were tabulated over a 20-year period! The alleged fatalities attributed to food supplements, which are mainly unconfirmed telephone reports, would amount to just 4 cases per year. For comparison, far more people succumb from bleeding gastric ulcers due to chronic aspirin ingestion.

If vitamin supplements produce serious side effects there is always legal recourse for consumers via product liability insurance. Health authorities continue to deride vitamin supplement manufacturers and irresponsibly frighten the public away from these beneficial products. By law, food supplements must be pure (free of contaminants), must not be misbranded, are subject to labelling laws and cannot make claims they prevent, cure or treat any disease. The Food & Drug Administration has enforcement authority to conduct inspections, issue warning letters, seize impure or misbranded products and pursue criminal action when indicated. Despite news reports to the contrary, the food supplement industry is not unregulated.

The Food & Drug Administration also does an about face

Not only has the American Medical Association made a U-turn concerning vitamins, during the writing of this book the Food & Drug Administration has announced an historic redirection. A new initiative will now encourage the flow of high-quality, science-based information regarding the health benefits of foods and food supplements. In its history, the FDA has only authorized three health claims for dietary supplements, all three being issued in recent years. These health claims are for folic acid in the prevention of birth defects, B vitamins to reduce the risk of blood vessel disease and omega-3 oils to reduce the risk of coronary heart disease.

< 14 >

Obviously responding to public demand, the new direction by the FDA opens the door for responsible parties to submit applications for health claims that can be affixed to product labels. It's possible that consumers may see claims that supplemental vitamin C prevents cataracts, folic acid prevents mental depression and Alzheimer's disease, vitamin C and vitamin B6 normalize blood pressure, vitamin E as alpha tocopherol, gamma tocopherol and tocotrienols, lycopene and vitamin D reduce the risk of prostate cancer.

When the weight of scientific evidence warrants, a health claim will be granted. Previously the FDA limited health claims to simple assertions, such as a particular food being a *good source of calcium.*" The FDA now recognizes that consumers *"are more likely to respond to information concerning the health benefits of consuming particular foods or supplements if the information identifies, with specificity, the health benefit associated with the product."* [FDA bulletin, Dec. 18, 2002]

> **Sometimes vitamin pills don't work for good reasons**

What may still be confusing to consumers is that while a health claim may now be printed on a food supplement label, the following statement must also accompany the health claim: *"This statement has not been evaluated by the Food & Drug Administration. This product is not intended to diagnose, treat, cure, or prevent any disease."* Obviously, the above precautionary statement may also need reevaluation. In fact, the FDA would have evaluated a health claim which would run contrary to the phrase *"This statement has not been evaluated by the FDA."*

The courts have ruled that health claims have a right under the First Amendment to the Constitution to be printed on product labels when proven by the weight of the scientific evidence to be true. While it has taken eight years to obtain this right, the FDA appears to be ready and willing to receive authoritative health claims that can be printed on product labels.

< 15 >

Relatively safe, but do they deliver health?

Then there is the issue of efficacy. Do vitamin supplements work, do they deliver on their promise of improved health? Are Americans just wasting their money on snake oil remedies?

Sometimes dosage on the label doesn't match what's inside the pills

Multivitamins certainly do deliver on the promise of improved health. Here is some of the evidence:

A combination of 1000 mcg of folic acid, 400 mcg of vitamin B12 and 10 mg of vitamin B6 has been shown to reduce undesirably high homocysteine levels and reversed narrowing of blood vessels. [New Eng J Med 345: 1593-1600, 2001]

The use of supplemental antioxidant vitamins C (1000 mg) and E (1000 IU) administered by intravenous or nasal/gastric tube significantly reduced the risk of lung problems and organ failure among hospitalized trauma patients and shortened their length of stay. Hospitals may soon be employing vitamins in their intensive care units. [Annals Surgery 236: 814-22, 2002]

Long-term supplementation with a multivitamin is also reported to have reduced the risk of colon cancer. [Ann Int Med 129: 517-24, 1998] Two other studies serve to confirm that protection from colon cancer provided by multivitamins, which is mostly attributed to their folic acid content. [Cancer Epidemiol Biomark Prev 6: 769-74, 1997; 11: 227-34, 2002]

Long-term use of multivitamins is associated with a reduced risk for cataracts, a blinding eye condition that universally affects all humans if they live long enough. [Am J Ophthalmology 132: 19-26, 2001]

Sometimes multivitamins don't work for good reasons. For instance, chronic use of water pills to control blood pressure helps wash out B

< 16 >

vitamins and may increase homocysteine levels. [Southern Medical J 92: 866-70, 1999] Millions of adults who take water pills to control blood pressure may not experience the full benefit of multivitamins.

Another study involving 47,152 female nurses suggests long-term usage of multivitamins does not prevent cataracts. But when smokers were removed from the study it became apparent multivitamins did significantly reduce cataract risk. [Epidemiology 10: 679-84, 1999] Smokers have higher needs for vitamin C and lutein than non-smokers and a shortage of these nutrients is linked with cataract formation. A larger dose of vitamin C and lutein than provided in most multivitamins may prevent cataracts. Additionally, the dosage of vitamin C is usually too low in common multivitamins to realize a protective effect from cataracts in non-smoking healthy adults.

> *Too much or too little riboflavin may cause cataracts*

Confuse the public: vitamin C

Consumers stand confused over the frequent contradictory headlines in the news concerning vitamins. For example, one day vitamin C is a wonder vitamin, the next day's news story says vitamin C could damage genetic material and promote cancer. Worldwide headlines recently advised the public to avoid more than 200 milligrams of vitamin C in food supplements when a test-tube study published in Science magazine errantly reported that mega-dose vitamin C may promote cancer by causing mutations in genetic material. [Science 292: 2083-86, 2001] A published rebuttal letter to the editors of Science magazine from this author pointed out that there were five recent human studies that used up to 10,000 milligrams of vitamin C which could not find any evidence of DNA damage. [Science 293:1993-5, 2001] No corrective news stories followed.

Actually, a news report issued two years prior also mistakenly alleged vitamin C could actually damage DNA. [Nature, April 9, 1998] But

< 17 >

that report was quickly refuted as well. Imagine the non-sensical nature of these news reports in light of the fact most animals (but not modern humans) naturally produce their own vitamin C, up to more than 13,000 milligrams per day, with no evidence of DNA mutation or increased risk of cancer. Americans need more vitamin C if for no

Mass use of multivitamins would reduce health care costs

other reason than the gastric tract of about half of the US adult population is infected with Helicobacter pylori which substantially reduces the availability of vitamin C. [Eur J Gastro Hepatol 13: 233-37, 2001] Some of these negative news stories appear to be intentionally designed to scare the public away from vitamin supplements.

Vitamin C has received its unfair share of biased or brazenly mistaken news reports. Another study reported that adults who took 500 milligrams of vitamin C per day experienced a 2.5 times greater thickening of the carotid (neck) arteries. [Presentation, American Heart Assn, March 2000] The researchers were unaware that vitamin C increases collagen production and strengthens the walls of arteries. High-dose vitamin C wasn't clogging neck arteries as reported, it was preventing disease. This, like many other negative reports on vitamins, was never published in a medical journal where it would have had to undergo peer review. But news agencies gave this story front-page placement.

Another common myth is that vitamin C causes kidney stones. Doctors frequently ask their patients with kidney stones if they are taking vitamin C and suggest they discontinue its use. Scientific studies do not confirm that vitamin C causes kidney stones, but myths have a way of never dying. [J Urology 155: 1847-51, 1996; Ann Nutrition Met 41: 269-82, 1997; J Am Soc Neph 10: 840-45, 1999; Journal Urology 151: 834-37, 1994]

< 18 >

Bad science

Then there is simply bad science being reported. For example, a recently published study reported that the provision of 200 milligrams of vitamin E increased the severity of respiratory infections among senior adults. [J Am Med Assn 288: 715-21, 2002] But vitamin E is a totally inappropriate nutrient to treat respiratory infection and it is only problematic because it competes with vitamin A for absorption. There is an increased need for vitamin A during bouts of infection. Another study suggested that vitamins C and E increased mortality rates from cardiovascular disease and coronary heart disease among low-risk American physicians who regularly supplemented their diet with these nutrients. [Archives Int Med 162: 1472-76, 2002] However, upon review, the authors of the report admit there was no proven association between mortality and the use of vitamin supplements and that actually there was a statistically significant reduced risk for fatal cardiovascular and coronary heart disease (34-41 percent) among a subset of users who employed both vitamins together. [Archives Int Med 162: December 9, 2002]

Vitamins and minerals protect DNA

Two studies were conducted on the combined cholesterol lowering properties of statin drugs combined with niacin (vitamin B3). The drug/B vitamin combination effectively lowered total and LDL *"bad"* cholesterol as well as triglycerides. But when supplemental antioxidants such as vitamin C and E were added to the statin drug/niacin regimen, the reduction in cholesterol was blunted. This led researchers to mistakenly claim that supplemental antioxidants simply have no place in the treatment of cardiovascular disease. [Arteriosclerosis Thrombosis Vascular Biology 21: 1320-26, 2001; New England Journal Medicine 345: 1583-92, 2001] These studies mischaracterize antioxidants. The statin drug and niacin combination impair liver function, may elevate liver enzyme levels which requires repeated testing, can induce muscle soreness and a muscle disorder that can be mortal, whereas the antioxidants were protecting the liver and preventing the toxicity caused

< 19 >

by the drugs. Modern medicine needs to employ methods to reduce cholesterol and prevent heart and blood vessel disease without agents that are toxic to the liver, such as tocotrienols, fish oil, allicin from garlic, lecithin and magnesium.

There are so many antagonists to vitamins, pharmaceutical companies who see them as a threat to prescription drugs, doctors who have been trained to view vitamins as *"snake oil"* and potentially hazardous, and nutritionists who fear vitamin pills will be used to replace a nutritious diet, that it's difficult for the scientific findings to get through to the public. Health care providers filter news stories about the health benefits of vitamins, often discounting or disqualifying well-founded scientific facts.

Physicians prescribe drugs that carry with them a long list of serious side effects, but warn patients away from essential vitamins as if they were toxic. On the other hand there are the zealots, those who have little knowledge of their use, but whose profit motives or personal experiences cause them to portray vitamins as *"magic bullets"* or *"cure-alls."*

Watchdog groups prove vitamins are oftentimes impotent

Watchdog groups have sprung up to check on the label claims on bottles of multivitamins. Consumerlab.com is one such organization that has revealed one of the common short-comings of vitamin supplements, the amount of nutrients provided often differs from the label. It's become apparent that vitamin supplement manufacturers may take shortcuts in order to better compete on the basis of price in the marketplace. In a published study various brands of vitamin E supplements varied from -41 percent to +57 percent of the labeled dosage. [J Urology 168: 150-54, 2002] This is a stain on the food supplement manufacturers. Companies that produce multivitamins are going to have to make greater efforts to ensure their products are properly labeled and that the amounts on the label match the actual amounts found in pills.

< 20 >

Vitamins: sometimes more trouble than benefit

One of the confounding revelations to this author have been the frequent phone calls from avid users of multivitamins who are completely unaware that poorly designed supplements they use may be an unrecognized factor in symptoms or even diseases they experience. Cataracts, sudden death heart attack, increased risk for infection, worsening of symptoms of arthritis and elevation of cholesterol may actually be induced by innocent-looking but poorly designed multivitamin pills.

The first time I became aware that vitamins aren't always helpful was when I assisted researchers in a clinical study at the Veterans Hospital system. Men with retinal problems who took a potent antioxidant formula for the eyes experienced no further progression of their retinal disease, but incurred a slight increased incidence of cataracts. How could this be?

It took some time to search through medical references to find that riboflavin, an essential B vitamin, prevents cataracts, but when taken in high doses (more than 10 milligrams) can actually be counter-productive and cause cataracts.

As reported by this author, vitamin studies often don't produce positive results because the wrong nutrients are being studied, because of poor dosage or lack of balance in a multivitamin formula. In a 5.5-year study of 83,639 male physicians in the US, of whom only 24.6 percent used multivitamins on a daily basis, there was no decrease in mortality from cardiovascular or coronary heart disease among multivitamin users. [Arch Intern Med 162: 1472-76, 2002] The problem here is that the type of vitamins being used by physician is not fully disclosed. US physicians likely take the run-of-the-mill multivitamins which the American Medical Association says is all that is needed to make up for nutritional gaps in the American diet.

Hence my conclusion, that consumers are unknowingly left in a quandary. Without accurate information from health care providers, and lacking well-designed brands of multivitamins to choose from,

< 21 >

how are health-minded Americans going to obtain the health benefits provided by vitamin supplements?

Failing health care system

In the midst of all this confusion there is turmoil in the American health care system. Health care plans and Medicare are going bankrupt. A growing population of retirees has forced politicians to cut back on health benefits in order to stave off the complete collapse of Medicare. The only way to keep health care costs from bankrupting the entire country is to lower the incidence of disease. An urgent report issued by the National Academy of Sciences says *"the American health care system is confronting a crisis"* and the delivery system is *"incapable of meeting the present, let alone future, needs of the American public."* The cost of health insurance is rising by 12 percent per year. [NY Times Nov 20, 2002]

In 1988 only 0.003 percent of US health dollars went toward prevention, a figure which hasn't changed significantly over the past decade. Health care providers aren't directing their patients to the health benefits provided by nutritional supplements, and when they do, they appear to recommend products that are not in keeping with the latest scientific reports.

The massive daily use of multivitamins has been proposed as a method of getting health care costs under control. For example, the National Defense Council Foundation indicates the federal government would save up to $6.3 billion annually by the provision of vitamin supplements to retired military personnel. If all Americans took a multivitamin the number of hospitalizations would be expected to drop and the insurance industry would save an estimated $5.5 billion (1995 dollars), which would result in lower insurance rates. [Managed Care Interface 11: 95-99, 1998] A report in the *Western Journal of Medicine* suggests vitamin supplements would reduce hospital costs by $20 billion annually.

< 22 >

Recommended daily allowance for genetic stability

Researchers have determined that shortages of vitamins and minerals, such as folic acid, vitamin B12, vitamin C, vitamin E or zinc, mimic the same damage caused to living cells by atomic radiation. The percentage of the US population that has a low intake of these nutrients ranges from 2 to 20 percent. Approximately 10 percent of the population has a folic acid deficiency that could induce chromosome breaks. This can lead to colon cancer. The quarter of the population that eats the fewest fruits and vegetables (5 servings a day is advised) experiences double the cancer rate when compared to groups with the highest plant food consumption. [Mutation Research 475: 7-20, 2001] Currently the focus of food fortification and supplemental vitamins is to prevent deficiency diseases like scurvy, pellagra, rickets and beri beri. But there may need to be a shift in thinking. Degenerative diseases and aging are partly caused by DNA damage. Instead of providing the minimum amount of nutrients to prevent deficiency diseases it may be time to think of providing the optimal amount to protect DNA. Recommended Daily Allowances for *genomic stability* have been proposed. [Food Chemistry Toxicology 40: 1113-17, 2002] Micronutrients and genomic stability: a new paradigm for recommended dietary allowances (RDAs).

For example, a study conducted by the National Center for Toxicological Research reveals that foods commonly contain components called heterocyclic amines that are mutagenic (induce abnormalities in genes) and produce tumors in laboratory animals under experimental conditions. The provision of vitamins C, E and beta carotene, alone or together, reduced *mutagenic frequency,* with vitamin E being the most protective. [Nutrition & Cancer 43: 103-10, 2002]

In another example, high-dose folic acid could inhibit cancer at the molecular genetic level since it is required for the production and repair of DNA. [FASEB J 12: 1491-97, 1998] Deficient levels of folic acid and vitamin B12 are associated with chromosome damage and a high concentration of homocysteine in the blood. A study was conducted with 700 mcg folic acid in fortified food or 2000 mcg in a

< 23 >

food supplement resulted in improved folic acid levels. It takes as long as 4 months to achieve saturation of folic acid in red blood cells after taking high-doses of this vitamin. It may take 2 months before folic acid therapy reduces chromosome abnormalities. Low-normal levels of vitamin B12 are related to increased rate of chromosome damage. The incidence of premature aging is related to genetic damage. The level of folic acid to eliminate deficiency disorders is not necessarily the same level required to prevent age-related diseases and to minimize genetic damage. Folic acid food fortification or supplementation decreases homocysteine levels by about 11 percent but does not have a significant impact on the genetic damage rate of chromosomes. The concentration of vitamin B12 required to prevent chromosome damage appears to be considerably higher than what would be considered sufficient levels of this vitamin. [Carcinogenesis 18: 1329-36, 1997] Genetic stability is achieved when the concentration of folic acid and vitamin B12 exceed the current recommended intake levels, that is, more than 400 micrograms of folic acid and 2 micrograms of vitamin B12. It is estimated that at least 700 micrograms of folic acid and 7 micrograms of vitamin B12 would be appropriate to achieve stability of DNA in young adults. [Mutation Research 475: 57-67, 2001]

The control and removal (chelation) of excess iron in the body is also important to remove the primary rusting agent in the body that has the potential, when released from binding proteins, to damage tissues and DNA. [Mutation Research 519: 151, 2002] Iron-binding nutrients known as bioflavonoids (citrus, quercetin, cranberry, blueberry, milk thistle) and from whole grains (IP6 rice bran extract) bind and remove iron efficiently.

The ends of DNA, called teleomeres, begin to shorten with advancing age which limits the number of times that cells renew themselves without causing mutations. Antioxidants can protect against teleomere loss and increase the number of times that have already been demonstrated to protect the DNA in experiments conducted with dogs. [J Nutrition 132: 1720S, 2002]

< 24 >

Rating the brands of multivitamins

The issue of ethics in health reporting has become an issue in recent times. Even prestigious medical journals have been criticized for publishing reports without full disclosure of authors' alliances with commercial interests. Let me say this at the top of the book, this author is attempting to provide you, the reader, with the best available science on this subject so you can analyze it for yourself. My job is to simplify and synopsize so you can get to the heart of the matter quickly. Even though I am called upon by various companies to tout their products from time to time, these commercial relationships cannot alter published scientific findings. Legal counsel advises me to provide authoritative references for all the statements made in this book and to recommend three or more sources for multivitamins, otherwise this book becomes nothing but veiled advertising.

This book draws a line in the sand. It does no good to provide raw information without actually ranking the brands of multivitamins for consumers. Without such a ranking most consumers would never be able to determine the value of the multivitamins available. There are simply too many factors to consider.

This 3rd multivitamin survey compares 25 key factors in brands of multivitamins regarding dosage, form of nutrient, balance, completeness and delivery. Once again our survey reveals that consumers can purchase well-designed multivitamins at far less cost than some of the exotic brands. Sadly, still most brands of multivitamins fall short of the mark. Many people will be disheartened to find that their favorite multivitamin didn't received a high rating. That's what this book is all about, to help urge manufacturers to make better products and to guide consumers to the best products available.

– Bill Sardi

< 25 >

Vitamin Truth #1
What's Wrong with Multivitamins

Mary develops cataracts- Were her cataracts caused by her vitamin pills?

For the past 10 years Mary Patterson has been taking a daily multivitamin with beta carotene providing 50,000 units of vitamin A activity, and she began juicing with beta carotene-rich carrot juice each morning when she heard that beta carotene might help prevent cancer. Mary's mother died an early death because of cancer and Mary wanted to protect herself. On her last trip to the eye doctor, 47-year old Mary was told she has cataracts developing in both eyes, which is about 25 years sooner than most adults. Mary ate fresh fruits and vegetables, exercised regularly and didn't smoke tobacco or drink alcohol, so she had no idea why she was developing cataracts. Actually, by overloading her diet with beta carotene, to the exclusion of other important protective plant pigments such as lutein and zeaxanthin, Mary has been hastening the day she would be diagnosed with cataracts. Read more below.

Edward's high cholesterol can't be lowered with drugs or diet. Did his vitamin pill cause this problem?

Edward Franklin has been taking 80 mg of zinc in a daily vitamin formula designed for people with eye problems. At about the same time Edward began taking vitamins, he developed high cholesterol (high LDL "bad" cholesterol), which prompted his doctor to recommend special diets and exercise. When those measures failed, cholesterol-lowering drugs were prescribed at $100 per month. Nothing seemed to work. Examination of Edward's vitamin regimen found that excessive amounts of zinc may impair the absorption and availability of copper, which can

< 26 >

result in elevated cholesterol readings. Once Edward reduced his daily zinc consumption his cholesterol fell to normal levels.

Susan follows advice to avoid osteoporosis but can't shake a variety of other health problems

Since Susan Meyer's grandmother has osteoporosis and has fallen and broken a hip, she doesn't want to fall victim to the same fate. A recent bone scan reveals Susan's bones are a bit thin for her age. Following advice from government health authorities, Susan begins taking 1500 mg of calcium daily and drinking more milk products. Within months Susan begins to experience recurrent migraines, uncontrollable eyelid twitches, fatigue, backaches, kidney stones and heart spasms. Two years later Susan is diagnosed with calcifications on her heart valves (mitral valve). Her doctor placed her on calcium-blocking drugs which cost about $100 per month. Susan is never advised that her calcium-magnesium ratio is way out of balance and may be the root cause of these health problems. Should Susan be taking that much calcium?

Why won't Bill's vitamin E pills stop his angina?

Bill Smothers takes a multivitamin pill that provides 60 units of vitamin E to help prevent recurrent angina. Bill doubles up on his multivitamin, taking two pills per day. But Bill's angina remains about the same. What Bill doesn't know is that he is taking synthetic vitamin E, which is only about one-third as potent as natural-source vitamin E. By doubling up on his multivitamin pill, Bill consumes excessive amounts of zinc, copper and iron, which only exacerbate his circulation problems.

< 27 >

Jonathan's multivitamin provides three times the daily requirement for vitamin C. So why does Jonathan exhibit signs of vitamin C deficiency?

Jonathan White takes a multivitamin pill that provides 120 mg of vitamin C, which is three times the Recommended Daily Allowance. From time to time Jonathan exhibits signs of skin bruising, bleeding gums, swelling at the back of his eyes, all which are symptoms of vitamin C deficiency. What Jonathan doesn't know is that he isn't getting enough vitamin C, and the type of vitamin C his multivitamin provides is incomplete.

< 28 >

History of Vitamins

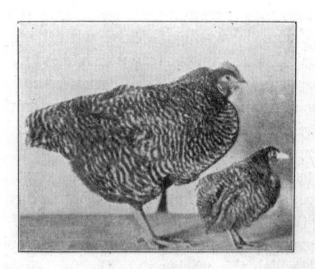

FIG. 8. SEVEN MONTHS OLD CHICKENS

Casimir Funk, 1884–1967, American biochemist, wrote the first book on vitamins and coined the term vitamines, which were essential substances in food to maintain health. [The Vitamines. Baltimore: Williams & Wilkins, 1922] The picture above is from Funk's book which shows the first documented evidence of the power of vitamins. The two chicks shown are seven months of age, but the chicken on the left was supplied a diet fortified with B vitamins.

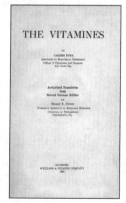

< 29 >

Vitamin Truth #2
Everybody Should Take Vitamins

The days of saying that a balanced diet will provide all the nutrients required to maintain health are over. A healthy diet is vital but a plethora of recently published studies show Americans can't achieve optimal health benefits from their diet alone. Vitamin supplements are essential today. Even the American Medical Association has finally recommended every American needs to take multivitamins based upon the realization that few Americans consume the recommended five servings of fruits and vegetables daily.

According to a University of California at Los Angeles study, <u>the daily consumption of 300 mg or more of vitamin C will add six years to a person's life.</u> [Newsweek, May 18, 1992; Epidemiology 3: 194-202, 1992] Harvard researchers report about the same amount of vitamin C reduces the risk of cataracts by 77-83 percent. [Am J Clinical Nutrition 66: 911-16, 1997] But as was the case with vitamin E, the amount of food needed to obtain this much vitamin C is impractical— requiring consumption of about five oranges a day.

The best diet will not produce optimal health

A 1993 report published in the _Journal of the American Medical Association_ reveals that the destructive process of oxidation (rusting of cells), caused by what are called free radicals, is involved in <u>all</u> human diseases, thus making antioxidants the antidotes to all disease. [J Am Medical Assn 270: 2024, 1993] Bruce Ames, noted biochemist at the University of California at Berkeley, writes that only 9 percent of Americans eat the recommended five servings of antioxidant-rich fruits and vegetables and that food supplements may be advisable. (A list of antioxidants is provided later in this book). Ames says the Recommended Daily Allowances for vitamin C and vitamin E _"are not_

< 30 >

adequate." [Proceedings Natl Academy Science 90: 7915-22, 1993] A review of the medical literature indicates antioxidant vitamins in food supplements are *"remarkably well tolerated and free from toxicity."* [Drug Safety 13: 8-14, 1995] Six milligrams or more of lutein, a yellow plant pigment, will cut in half the risk of developing a blinding eye disease in the later years of life (macular degeneration).

Both folic acid and lutein are available in dark-green leafy vegetables such as kale and spinach, which would have to be consumed daily to achieve optimal levels of these nutrients. In the real world however, less than 10 percent of the population actually consumes plant foods on a regular basis.

Other recent studies show that up to 37 percent of American adults are deficient in vitamin D, a nutrient that helps to prevent brittle bones (osteoporosis) and cancer. [New England Journal Medicine 338: 777-83, 1998]

Up to 1 million American adults do not properly absorb vitamin B12, a problem which can lead to symptoms of fatigue, short-term memory loss and nerve disorders. Blood tests do not always uncover a B12 deficiency. In a country that is well nourished in calories, nutritional deficiencies abound.

Nutrient deficiencies don't stop with vitamins. Mineral deficiencies are also common. According to a newly published report from *the National Academy of Sciences*, about 8 out of 10 Americans fall short by about 100-200 mg of their daily requirement for magnesium. [Dietary Reference Intakes, National Academy Press, 1997] This mineral deficiency is directly associated with sudden death heart attack, cases of asthma, allergies, migraines, high blood pressure, kidney stones and heart valve calcifications. An estimated 420 adults succumb to sudden death heart attack every day in America due to a lack of magnesium.

The average American consumes about 10 mg of elemental zinc from the diet. Nearly all Americans fall short of the suggested daily intake of zinc

< 31 >

(15 mg). The type of zinc in foods is not easily absorbed. Zinc, in the right amount, is required to produce enzymes within the body and to maintain a healthy immune system. The sense of taste and smell depend upon adequate intake of zinc.

Americans consume only about 80 mcg of daily selenium, a trace mineral that has been shown to significantly reduce the risk of viral infections, cancer and heart disease. [J Am Medical Assn. 276: 1957-63, 1996] While most Americans get adequate amounts of this trace mineral, experts indicate health parameters would improve if they consumed 200-400 micrograms per day of organic selenium. Too many Americans live in selenium-poor soil areas and are thus unable to get enough of this trace mineral from food. Many health authorities suggest Americans consume 200 mcg of selenium daily. It is interesting that all farm animals in Britain are administered selenium supplements because of obvious health benefits, but humans in Britain are not. [British Medical Journal 314: 387-88, 1997]

There is additional evidence that multivitamins are beneficial. Older American adults who took a multivitamin tablet providing 18 different nutrients for a year experienced only 18 sick days versus 32 days for adults who did not take vitamins. [The Lancet 340: 1124-27, 1992] It was recently found that the need for cataract surgery is reduced by 25 percent among multivitamin users. [American Journal Public Health 84: 788-92, 1994] When 129 healthy young adults consumed 9 vitamins in dosages 10 times greater than the Recommended Daily Allowance, their mood improved. [Neuropsychobiology 32: 98-105, 1995]

Dr. Bruce Ames recently told an audience of researchers at a conference of the Society of Toxicology that *"nutrient deficiency may explain why the quarter of the population that eats the fewest fruits and vegetables has double the cancer rate of the quarter that eats the most fruits and vegetables…. I'm convinced that if we got a multivitamin-mineral pill into the poor, we'd have an enormous increase in health."* Ames contends that vitamin formulas should be well designed because too many vitamins can be as bad as too

< 32 >

few. For example, most men already get too much iron, he says. [Lack of Vitamins May Cause Cancer, Reuters, October 28, 1998]

A Tufts University study shows that Americans in low income groups eat as much food as richer groups, but their diets are lower in vitamins. Ames says the poor are eating such vitamin-deficient diets they are battering their DNA, causing cancer and maybe damaging their brains. Ames says when the populace hears that chemicals or pesticide residues cause cancer it distracts from the real problem — a lack of antioxidant nutrients. He says that antioxidants prevent damage to DNA within cells that causes cancer.

> **Expect fewer sick days taking a multivitamin**

"If you don't get enough vitamins C and E, it is like irradiating yourself," says Dr. Ames. It's very difficult to get anyone to change their diet to include five servings of fresh fruits and vegetables a day. *"You can solve all these problems with a multivitamin pill,"* says Ames. [Reuters June 20, 2000] Just adding up these nutritional deficiencies is enough to prompt every American to consider taking a daily multivitamin, as good health insurance.

Consumer Reports says *"Millions of people with subtle deficiencies might benefit from taking a daily multivitamin/mineral supplement,"* and that *"even people who get recommended levels of vitamins and minerals may not be getting enough for optimal health."* [Consumer Reports 59: 560-69, 1994] With all of this evidence, how many Americans actually take a multivitamin pill?

Out of a population of 275+ million Americans, an estimated 115 million periodically take vitamin supplements of any kind, but only about a third, 86.5 million, are regular users. Many of the health benefits reported in published studies were only apparent among those who took vitamins for many years, rather than just occasionally.

< 33 >

Even then, <u>most vitamin users only purchase singular nutrients, like vitamin C or vitamin E, rather than a good daily multivitamin</u>. This is probably because most consumers hear about the health benefits of vitamins one at a time.

<u>One survey indicates 41 percent of older Americans who take vitamin supplements take only a single nutrient and just 10 percent take vitamin supplements that provide 7 or more nutrients</u>. [J Am Dietetic Association 90: 671-76, 1990] In another survey, 26 percent of adults took vitamin supplements, 71 percent who only took one nutrient. [Pharmacology 16: 715-20, 1996]

A survey of 200 consecutive patients attending a medical clinic reveals that 52 percent had consumed at least one vitamin supplement in the past 12 months, while only 18 percent took 2-5 nutrients and 3 percent took 6-13 nutrients. [J Am Board Family Practice 9: 249-53, 1996]

To make up for dietary deficiencies, health-minded consumers should consume an array of B vitamins, about ten minerals, the four fat-soluble vitamins (A,D,E,K), plus antioxidants like vitamin C, beta carotene and lutein, most which are essential for life. Buying and consuming a bottle of each of these nutrients would be tedious and expensive, so multivitamins are convenient and economical.

<u>Bottom line</u>: Take multivitamins to help make up for the many nutritional deficiencies in the American diet and to achieve optimal health benefits such as reduced risk of heart attack, cataracts and cancer.

< 34 >

Vitamin Truth #3
The Recommended Daily Allowance
Is Obsolete

Visually scan the label on a bottle of multivitamins. Look where it says percentage of <u>daily value</u>. Consumers are frequently misled when they read that the multivitamin they are taking provides 100 percent of the Daily Value (DV), or the Recommended Daily Allowance (RDA) or the new Reference Daily Intake (RDI).

These confusing acronyms may lull health-conscious consumers into falsely believing products that provide 200 percent or 300 percent or even 3000 percent more than the DV, RDA or RDI are a waste of money or even more disconcerting, may be an overdose. FDA law requires nutrients in multivitamins to be labelled as a percentage of the Daily Value, but these amounts are just enough to prevent deficiencies, not produce optimal health. [Nutrition Reviews 52: 266-70, 1994]

Typical dietary intake + a common multivitamin is still not adequate

Poorly formulated multivitamins plus the average diet don't provide the amount of nutrients found in five servings of fruits and vegetables.

Even the recommended five servings of fresh fruits and vegetables, which only a small percentage of Americans consume, would provide up to 6 mg of beta carotene, 225 mg of vitamin C and 23-27 IU of vitamin E. Now look at the chart below and you will notice that <u>the typical dietary intake of nutrients plus the amount provided by many brands of multivitamins is not equivalent to the amount provided by five servings of fresh plant foods</u>.

< 35 >

5-servings of fresh fruits and vegetables provides	Typical Amt in dime-a-day multivitamins	Typical Dietary intake	Shortage
Vitamin C 225 mg	60-90 mg	110 mg	35-55 mg
Vitamin E 23-27 IU	15 IU	10 IU	0-2 IU
Beta carotene 6 mg 20,000 IU Vitamin A activity	3 mg 10,000 IU	.75 mg 2500 IU	2.25 mg 7500 IU
Lutein/ zeaxanthin 5000-6000 mcg spinach and kale	500 mcg Usually none	2314 mcg	2200-3200 mcg

What weak multivitamins do provide are the Recommended Daily Allowances, now recognized as outdated by many nutritionists.

If you are….

A growing child,
Pregnant or lactating,
Under physical or emotional stress,
Participate in regular physical exercise,
Smoke tobacco,
Consume excessive alcohol,
Are exposed to toxic chemicals,
Overweight,
Take certain medications,
Have digestive problems,
Regularly consume fast foods or junk foods,
Or you are over age 70 or have a chronic health problem like diabetes or high blood pressure,
… then you will need to consume more than the Recommended Daily Allowance (or the new Reference Daily Intake).

< 36 >

Decades ago, the Recommended Daily Allowance (RDA) was developed to determine the minimal amount of certain nutrients required to prevent deficiency diseases like pellagra (niacin), scurvy (vitamin C), rickets (vitamin D), beri beri (vitamin B1-thiamin), night blindness (vitamin A), growth problems (vitamin E) and birth defects (folic acid). Today, however, it is obvious that greater health benefits can be achieved by consuming more than the Recommended Daily Allowance.

Unfortunately, since there hasn't been much publicity about the limitations of the RDA, most consumers will read the labels on vitamin bottles and assume that 100 percent of the Recommended Daily Allowance is sufficient to maintain their health. This is a false assumption. Asks Robert D. Reynolds, PhD, from the Department of Nutrition and Medical Dietetics at the University of Illinois: *"Are the Recommended Daily Allowances (RDAs) only for healthy persons or should they also include those persons with some type of disease, as normally occurs in approximately 50 percent of the population at any given point in time?"* [J Am College Nutrition 13: 118-26, 1994] The 1989 RDA says *"Individuals with special nutritional needs are not covered by the RDAs."* So much for relying on labels printed on vitamin bottles.

Recently the National Institute of Medicine slightly increased the daily requirement for vitamin C from 60 to 75 milligrams. Yet the US Department of Agriculture and the National Cancer Institute recommend consumption of at least five servings of fresh fruits and vegetables, equaling 210-280 milligrams of vitamin C. The new Reference Daily Intake for vitamin C does not correlate with data on disease prevention.

< 37 >

Plant Foods You Should Be Eating	
Papaya	Provides twice the vitamin C as an orange 120 mg
Kiwi	Provides more vitamin C than papaya
Figs	Provides an excellent non-dairy source of calcium
Bananas	Makes up for shortage of potassium in the diet; about 475 mg potassium per banana; supplements limited to 99 mg
Spinach	Excellent source of lutein, calcium, magnesium
Kale	Provides twice the lutein/zeaxanthin as spinach
Tomatoes	Provides a more economical source of lycopene than supplements
Watermelon	A better source of lycopene than tomatoes
Onions	Excellent source of bioflavonoids (quercetin)
Berries, Cherries, Grapes	Other good sources of bioflavonoids
Broccoli	Provides sulfur compounds
Asparagus	Excellent source of sulfur

The best diet is not good enough

The decades physicians have advised the public that all the nutrients they need for health can be acquired from foods. The very best diet you can consume, loaded with fresh fruits and vegetables, will not provide your body with enough vitamin E (200 International Units) to maintain optimal immunity from infectious disease. [Methods Enzymology 282: 247-63, 1997] A person would need to eat 30 ounces of almonds (over 2500 calories) or ten tablespoons of wheat germ oil to get that much vitamin E. The amount of vitamin C obtained with a plant food-rich diet (~225 mg), is not enough to prevent age-related cataracts (300 mg), nor enough to maintain healthy blood pressure (500 mg), and is far short of the 2000+ milligrams of vitamin C the human body once produced naturally in the liver before a genetic mutation occurred centuries ago. A person would have to eat six oranges a day to get enough vitamin C

< 38 >

to prevent cataracts. The very best diet will not provide your body with enough folic acid to prevent age-related maladies such as brain and blood vessel disease. The best diet will not provide your body with enough vitamin B12 to eliminate the risk of short-term memory loss and nerve problems. The American diet does not provide a sufficient amount of magnesium to prevent sudden heart spasm. Multivitamin and mineral supplements are the best approach to health promotion.

< 39 >

SPECIAL NUTRITIONAL NEEDS OF THE AMERICAN POPULATION THAT CANNOT BE MET BY THE BEST DIET OR MOST MULTIVITAMINS

Total US Population: ~280 million

Athletes, exercisers: Untold millions. Exercise produces more oxidation within the body; countered by antioxidants. [Cell Biochem Function 16: 269-75, 1998] Antioxidant pills improve health parameters among athletes in training. [Int J Sports Med 21: 146-50, 2000]

Heart disease patients: 50+ million. Vitamin E may be beneficial. [Archives Family Medicine 8: 537-42, 1999]

Hypertensive patients: 43 million. 500 mg vitamin C daily reduces blood pressure similar to drugs. [The Lancet 354: Dec 1999]

Diabetics: 15.7 million. (798,000 new cases annually)
Vitamin E has protective effect.
[Am J Clinical Nutrition 63: 753-59, 1996]

Hospitalized: 33 million annually. Hospitalized have increased need for antioxidant nutrients. [Int Journal Vitamin Nutrition Research 54: 65-74, 1984]

Pregnant and lactating females: 4 million. US women give birth annually; offspring must obtain nutrients from mother. Fertile women require folic acid before conception to prevent birth defects.

Tobacco smokers: 66 million. Smokers require 25 mg vitamin C for each cigarette smoked. [Ann NY Academy Sciences 258: 156-67, 1975]

Elderly: 34 million. Older adults have increased nutritional needs. [Geriatric Nutrition, Raven Press 1998]

Retirees at risk for cataracts: 34 million. 10-year users of 250 mg vitamin C have 45-83 percent reduction in risk. [British Med J 305: 335-39, 1992]

< 40 >

Vitamin Truth #4
Make Certain Your Multivitamin Is Potent

OK, you've now learned that there are proven, valuable health benefits to be gained by taking a full range of vitamins, minerals and other nutrients. Trouble is, how do you choose the best from the bewildering array of products in stores? On your next trip to the supermarket or drug store you will have made a mental note to pick up a bottle of multivitamins, a brand that won't dent your pocketbook too much. One that provides a wide array of nutrients. Centrum, a popular brand of vitamins, provides 31 nutrients per pill. That should about do it, right? Well, maybe not.

In one survey, <u>eight out of ten vitamin supplement users only consumed the Recommended Daily Allowance, which would be insufficient to prevent many health problems</u>. [J Am Board Family Practice 9: 249-53, 1996]

The Alliance for Aging Research suggests that vitamin pills provide at least 250-1000 mg of vitamin C and 100-400 IU vitamin E. The University of California Berkeley *Wellness Letter* suggests 250-500 mg vitamin C and 200-400 units of vitamin E. [Berkeley Wellness Letter Sept. 1999] The most widely advertised daily multivitamins, One-A-Day, Centrum and Theragran, don't come close to providing these dosages of nutrients. Most Americans are taking vitamins that are impotent. These vitamin pills won't provide the levels of nutrients outlined in scientific studies to prevent disease and maintain good health.

The American Medical Association (AMA) has finally recommended multivitamins for everybody, but only those multivitamins minimal-dose brands. It's a contradiction to say that most Americans don't eat the recommended five servings of fruits and vegetables, therefore they need a low-dose multivitamin when a plant-food rich diet will provide about 225 mg of vitamin C while the dime-a-day multivitamins recommended

< 41 >

by the AMA only provide 60-90 mgs of vitamin C. A survey shows that 90 percent of the time pharmacists recommend Centrum, Theragran or a generic copy of these multivitamins. [American Druggist, Sept. 1997]

Get More Folic Acid
The folic acid revolution: supplements superior to food fortification

In just the last few years folic acid has risen to super-star status among vitamins. This inexpensive B vitamin is a nutritional antidote to premature aging and chronic age-related disease. Folic acid recently gained public attention for its ability to prevent birth defects (spina bifida). But now researchers recongize folic acid's health benefits extend far beyond this to prevent Alzheimer's disease, heart and

Americans need more folic acid than fortified foods provide

blood vessel disease and even colon cancer. Furthermore, folic acid food supplements appear to deliver on folic acid's health benefits more so than fortified foods. Researchers now suggest an optimal intake level of folic acid to protect against a variety of medical conditions. [Int J Vitam Nutr Res 72: 46-52, 2002] Researchers now report that older adults, in particular males over age 70, with low folic acid intake which correlates with high levels of an undesirable blood protein called homocysteine, are more likely to experience memory problems and elevated blood pressure. [J Am Geriatrics Society 50: 2014, 2002]

Folic acid, a B vitamin, reduces the risk of birth defects by 75 percent [J Am College Nutrition 13: 118-26, 1994] and the buildup of an undesirable protein in the blood stream (homocysteine) that causes strokes and heart attacks. [Annals Nutrition Metabolism 41: 331-43, 1997]

Our bodies use folic acid and choline to convert the potentially toxic amino acid homocysteine into another amino acid called methionine. Methionine then converts into S-adenosylmethionine (SAMe), which has

< 42 >

become a popular food supplement on its own as a natural antidepressant and anti-inflammatory agent. Homocysteine is extremely toxic to blood vessels resulting in disease, heart attacks and strokes. The body also needs sufficient levels of folic acid to produce choline, an amino acid required for the production of certain brain chemicals (acetycholine) involved in memory and blood pressure control. [ARS News March 2001]

How much folic acid to stop birth defects?

Folic acid is necessary for red blood cell production and neural tube formation

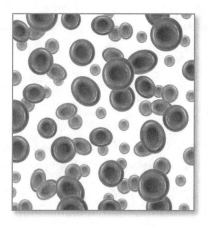
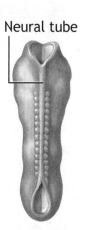

Neural tube

✿A.D.A.M.

In 1992 the US Public Health Service issued a recommendation that all women of childbearing age capable of becoming pregnant consume 400 mcg of folic acid a day in order to decrease the risk of having a baby with birth defects. [Morbidity Mortality Weekly Reports 41: 1-7, 1992] This was only the second approved health claim for a vitamin in 88 years. A decade earlier health officials had data in their hands which showed that a lack of folic acid was directly related to birth defects. Had a more timely action taken place to fortify foods and recommend folic acid supplements an estimated 13,000 birth defects could have been prevented yielding cost saving exceeding $5 billion. In 1996 the US Food & Drug Administration issued a regulation requiring that all

< 43 >

enriched cereal-grain products be fortified with folic acid by January of 1998. It was anticipated that food fortification would raise intake levels by about 100 micrograms, but it almost doubled intake levels (190 mcg).

Food-bound folic acid is not as bioavailable as in vitamin pills [J Nutrition 132: 2792-98, 2002] But this amount of folic acid was still found to be lacking. In 1999 it was estimated that 68-87 percent of US females of childbearing age had folic acid intakes below the 400 mcg point. [Am J Clin Nut 70: 198-207, 1999] About 80 percent of women take folic acid supplements once they realize they are pregnant. The neural tube closes 23 to 27 days after conception, so it is essential to begin supplementation prior to conception since optimal folic acid levels take a few weeks to achieve. Even spontaneous abortion is related to low folic acid levels. [J Am Med Assn 288: 1867-73, 2002]

A review of the amount of folic acid intake required to reduce birth defects is undergoing serious re-evaluation. Food fortification modestly reduces the risk by about 20 percent. Supplementation with 400 micrograms which has been found to reduce the risk for birth defects among fertile women by about 36 percent. The provision of 1000 micrograms would reduce risk by 57 percent and a whopping 5000 mcg by 85 percent. *"Women planning a pregnancy should take 5000 mcg folic acid tablets daily instead of the 400 microgram tablets presently recommended."* [The Lancet 358: 2069-73, 2001] The Centers for Disease Control now recommends women at high risk for birth defects in their offspring take 4000 mcg of folic acid from prior to conception through their first trimester to reduce risk. [MMWR Recomm Rep 51: 1-3, 2002] That's ten times more folic acid than most vitamin tablets provide.

Supplements outperform fortified foods

The bioavailability of folic acid from supplements is at least double that of dietary folic acid. [J Gender Specif Med 2: 24-28, 1999] In one study food fortification decreases the percentage of adults whose folic acid intake was below suggested levels from 48 percent to 7 percent. Among

< 44 >

adults who used supplements, only 1 percent remained below adequacy levels! [Morbidity Mortality Weekly Reports 41: 1-7, 1992]

A recent study showed that a pack-a-day smoking habit increased homocysteine levels by 18 percent. Elevated homocysteine levels in smokers were offset by high dietary intake of folic acid (green leafy vegetables) by 10-15 percent and reduced by 200 percent with folic acid supplements. So the supplements outperformed fortified foods. Researchers concluded that folic acid supplements can *"offset the effects of an unhealthy lifestyle."* [Int J Vitamin Nut Res 69: 322-29, 1999]

	Folic acid provided	Lower homocysteine
Folic acid supplement	437 mcg	21%
Fortified cereal	298 mcg	24%
Food (non-fortified)	418 mcg	9%
Am J Clin Nut 71: 448-54, 2000		
Folic acid supplements reduce undesirably high homocysteine levels better than foods.		

Just how much folic acid should be consumed?

Daily supplementation with 500 mcg of folic acid is expected to reduce homocysteine concentrations by about 25 percent and 500 mcg of vitamin B12 would further reduce homocysteine levels by another 7 percent. [British Med J 316: 894-98, 1998] Other researchers have determined that 650 mcg of folic acid is the minimum effective dose to reduce homocysteine. [Annals Pharm 34: 57-65, 2000]

Another study set out to determine the lowest supplemental dose of folic acid that would produce the maximum homocysteine reduction among adults with coronary artery disease. It was determined that 800 micrograms maximally reduced homocysteine. Researchers said *"it would be reasonable for clinicians to consider advising patients with heart disease to take 800 micrograms of folic acid each day,"* and that *"current US*

< 45 >

food fortification levels will achieve only a small proportion of the achievable homocysteine reduction. " [Archives Int Med 161: 695-700, 2001]

Dutch researchers used 5000 mcg (5 mg) of supplemental folic acid and found it reduced homocysteine levels by 40 percent. They suggest that the currently recommended intake of folic acid is insufficient to protect from disease. [Ned Tijdschr Geneeskd 142: 782-86, 1998]

Do folic acid supplements work?

Most physicians are waiting for studies to be completed. But a six-year study in Canada has already found that multivitamins with folic acid reduce the relative risk for coronary artery disease among men by 69 percent. Researchers said *"the study suggests that the reduced risk between vitamin supplement use and coronary artery disease is real."* [Clinical Cardiology 12: 930-34, 1996] A combination of 1000 mcg of folic acid, 400 mcg of vitamin B12 and 10 mg of vitamin B6 reduced homocysteine levels and reversed narrowing of blood vessels. [New Eng J Med 345: 1593-1600, 2001] Another study showed that among 80,082 women who had been taking an average of 696 mcg of folic acid and 4.6 mg of vitamin B6 reduced their relative risk for coronary heart disease by 31 percent. In women who consumed more than one alcoholic drink per day their risk for coronary heart disease was reduced by 73 percent. The report said: *"Intake of these vitamins above the recommended dietary allowance may be important in the primary prevention of coronary heart disease among women."* [J AM Med Assn 279: 359-64, 1998] One study showed the annual cost of medication for a patient with coronary artery disease is around $1250 of which insurance may pay around 65 percent of these costs, leaving about $436 in out-of-pocket costs. [J Am Board Family Practice 12: 200-05, 1999] Compare this to 800 mcg tablets of folic acid which would cost about $25 for a whole year's supply.

The provision of folic acid, vitamin B12 and vitamin B6 has been demonstrated to reduce adverse events after coronary or other blood vessel surgery. [J AM Med Assn 288: 973-79, 2002] In another study, the top dietary intake of folic acid, about 340 mcg per day, decreased the

< 46 >

relative risk of heart attack by 43 percent. [Epidemiology 13: 700-06, 2002]

At least three studies serve to confirm that protection from colon cancer provided by multivitamins, which is mostly attributed to their folic acid content. [Cancer Epidemiol Biomark Prev 6: 769-74, 1997; 11: 227-34, 2002; Ann Int Med 129: 517-24, 1998] High alcohol consumption, which has a strong effect at depleting folic acid, is associated with elevated risk for colon cancer. [J Nutrition 132: 2350-55S, 2002] A daily 2000 mcg folic acid supplement regimen has been employed to successfully reverse pre-cancerous polyps (adenomas) in the colon. [Gut 51: 195-99, 2002]

Use of multivitamins with folic acid during pregnancy reduce the risk of high blood pressure during pregnancy by 45 percent. [Am J Epidemiology 156: 806-12, 2002]

Folic acid supplements appear to be beneficial to the nervous system. Within one month the provision of folic acid (750 mcg), vitamin B12 (15 mcg), vitamin B6 (75 mg) was shown to have *a significant positive effect on some measures of memory performance.*" [J Nutrition 132: 1345-56, 2002]

A striking study, overlooked since 1982, reveals that a folic acid deficiency may sometimes result in the appearance of abnormal cells on a Pap smear. Apparently oral contraceptives reduce folic acid levels in females which can result in abnormal Pap tests, which are reversible with folic acid supplements. [Am J Clin Nut 35: 73-82, 1982] Papilloma viral infection, which is believed to be primary cause of cervical cancer, is less prevalent among women who have high red blood cell levels of folic acid. [Am J Obstet Gynecol 166: 803-09, 1992]

The use of high-dose folic acid supplements for major mental depression is very promising. Low vitamin levels are indicative of more severe depression. Blood folic acid levels may be considered to be normal in some of these cases. [J Am Ger Soc 39: 252-57, 1991] Among adults

< 47 >

90-101 years of age, the ability to recall words and objects was found to be related to their folic acid levels. [Biol Psychiatry 45: 1472-80, 1999] Beta amyloid peptide is believed to be a brain plaque involved in the onset of Alzheimer's disease. A study conducted at the National Institute on Aging Gerontology Research Center in Baltimore found that folic acid deficiency impairs the repair of nerve cells in the brain making them prone to damage caused by beta amyloid peptide. [J Neuroscience 22: 1752-62, 2002] Low intake of folic acid has now been linked to an increased risk for Alzheimer's disease. [New Eng J Med 346: 476-83, 2002]

High-dose folic acid may reduce mental depression

Folic acid shortages greater than estimated

Folic acid shortages may be much higher than the reported 30 percent among adults. [FASEB J 12: 1491-97, 1998] About 5 to 7 percent of the population (14-20 million people) carries a single copy of a gene for elevated homocysteine levels. People who carry this gene have homocysteine levels 2 to 4 times higher than normal. In a 1992 study showed that among 15,000 men whose homocysteine levels were just 12 percent above the high end of the normal range had a 300 percent increased risk of heart attack. [Ann Internal Med 130: 933-37, 1999] A significant percentage of the population with this genetic condition need far more folic acid than recommended daily intake levels. [NIH News Release, May 30, 1997]

What about overdose of folic acid?

Can you get too much folic acid? It's difficult to find any reports of adverse side effects from taking high-dose folic acid supplements other than this vitamin could mask a vitamin B12 deficiency. A 1997 report showed that just 10 of 308 adults ranging in age from 65 to 94 years took 800 mcg of supplemental folic acid. There were an additional 145 adults (47 percent) took 400 mcg folic acid from supplements. Dietary

< 48 >

consumption plus fortified foods provided an additional 348 mcg of folic acid, for a total folic acid intake from dietary and supplemental sources ranging from 748 to 1148 mcg. No side effects were noted. [J Am Diet Assn 97: 167-73, 1997]

Suggestions that high-dose folic acid supplements are unsafe appear to be weak and founded primarily on case reports, not actual studies. The primary concern is that mega-dose folic acid would mask a deficiency of vitamin B12. The remedy, obviously, is always to provide these two vitamins together in supplements. [Clin Biochem 33: 337-43, 2000] Some studies indicate vitamin B12 is as important or more important than folic acid in reducing elevated homocysteine levels. [Clin Cardiology 25: 495-501, 2002] This is another good reason to take multivitamins instead of individual supplements. Reviewers suggest folic acid in doses up to 5000 mcg are *"unlikely to cause adverse effects."* [Archives Internal Med 156: 1638-44, 1996]

Folic acid from foods- mean intake US adults	277 micrograms
Folic acid food fortification	190 micrograms
Folic acid from provided in most multivitamins	400 micrograms
Total folic acid intake all sources	867 micrograms

Bottom line: How much folic acid should be supplied in multivitamins? The diet, particularly green leafy vegetables, and fortified foods provides anywhere from 200-350 mcg of folic acid. But Americans have many practices that reduce folic acid and elevate undesirable homocysteine. Coffee, and to a lesser extent alcohol and tobacco, elevate homocysteine levels, which increases the need for folic acid. [Pharmacol Rev 54: 599-618, 2002] Certain medications deplete folic acid, such as diuretics (water pills) used to control high blood pressure, non-steroidal anti-inflammatory drugs such as aspirin and ibuprofen, some antibiotics (tetracyclines, mycins, cillins), antidiabetic drugs (Metformin-Glucophage), birth control pills and anti-heartburn acid blockers. The widespread use of the above agents increases the dosage of folic acid

< 49 >

that should be provided in food supplements. <u>Folic acid supplements are superior to food fortification as a strategy to reduce disease</u>. Since many fertile females do not take folic acid till they are pregnant, this underscores the need for supplemental folic acid. In light of the current knowledge on folic acid, <u>multivitamins should provide a minimum of 800 mcg of folic acid</u>. Any suggestion to provide more than 1000 micrograms of folic acid in food supplements will require approval by health authorities since supplements that exceed 1000 mcg must be sold on a prescription-only basis. Folic acid must be accompanied by vitamin B12 to eliminate instances were folic acid masks a B12 deficiency. The mass use of folic acid/vitamin B12 supplements would significantly reduce mortality rates, saving hundreds of thousands of lives over a 10-year period. [J Am Med Assoc 86: 936-43, 2001]

Get more vitamin B12

Even though many foods today are fortified with vitamins to prevent the common deficiency diseases, a <u>prevalent vitamin deficiency disease still exists</u> in the population at large that the best diet and even most multivitamin can't cure --- <u>pernicious anemia. Its symptoms are pervasive among senior adults, short-term memory loss, sore tongue, burning, tingling, numb feet.</u> [J Geron Biol Sci Med Sci 57: 583M, 2002] Other health problems are also linked to vitamin B12 deficiency.

- A shortage of vitamin B12 is linked to bladder control problems (incontinence) in older adults. [J Am Ger Soc 46: 931, 1998]

- Ringing in the ears (tinnitus) is associated with low B12 status. [Am J Otolaryngol 14: 94, 1993] Age-related hearing loss is another problem now linked to shortages of vitamin B12. [Am J Clin Nut 69: 564-71, 1999]

- Mental depression is associated with vitamin B12 deficiency. [Am J Psychiatry 157: 715-21, 2000]

< 50 >

These symptoms are often caused, not by a lack of vitamin B12, but the inability to absorb B12 from foods. An estimated 10 to 30 percent of older adults have lost their ability to absorb vitamin B12. [Am J Health Sys Pharm 55: 981, 1998] If 1 million Americans came down with beri beri there would be an immediate uproar to fortify foods with more vitamin B1 (thiamin). One report estimates there are 800,000 people who have undiagnosed and untreated pernicious anemia in the US. [Arch Int Med 156: 1097, 1996] Nearly a million American adults have vitamin B12 deficiency and little is done about the problem. In 1994 The Saturday Evening Post reported on one physician's then 33-year battle to raise the allowances for this vitamin. No action has been taken.

> **Vitamin B12 from foods and vitamin pills may be poorly absorbed**

Only about 1 percent of vitamin B12 is absorbed from foods by many older adults. The problem is that protein-bound vitamin B12 in foods is barely absorbed due to an enzyme shortage (pepsin) or lack of stomach acid. [Ann Rev Nut 19: 257-77, 1999] Even younger adults may have absorption problems. The U.S. Department of Agriculture says as much as 40 percent of the US adult population may be deficient in vitamin B12. [ARS News, August 2, 2000] B12 deficiency may remain undetected for long periods of time and may not be apparent by blood testing. The digestive tract of approximately 50 percent of the American adult population is infected with Helicobacter pylori, a bacterium that inhibits vitamin B12 absorption. [Arch Int Med 160: 1349, 2000]

Drugs such as the heartburn medications (histamine blockers Pepcid, Zantac, Tagamet, Prilosec, Nexium) and anti-diabetic drugs (Glucophage) may interfere with vitamin B12 absorption. [Drug Induced Nutrient Depletion Handbook, 2nd edition] Supplemental B12 should be taken by anyone on these drugs.

Vitamin B12 deficiency cannot be corrected by fortifying foods since the dosage required to correct the problem can only be achieved by vitamin supplements. High oral doses have been shown to be as effective as B12

< 51 >

injections. Supplements providing 25 mcg of vitamin B12 may help to reduce homocysteine levels. [J Am Geriatrics Soc 50: 1401, 2002] Provision of 25 and 100 mcg to older adults was not found to overcome deficiency. Only 7 of 20 adults given up to 100 mcg of vitamin B12 normalized their B12 levels. Another study indicates 50 mcg, but not 10 mcg, was effective in increasing blood serum levels of vitamin B12. [J Am Ger Soc 50: 146, 2002] One study suggests even as much as 1000 mcg of B12 from supplements is required to normalize adults. [J Am Geriatrics Society 50: 1789, 2002] Most daily multivitamin pills only provide the Recommended Daily Allowance, 6 mcg, but it takes 300-1000 micrograms in daily oral doses to eliminate the problem of pernicious anemia. [J Am Geriatric Soc 45: 122, 1997; Int J Vitam Nutr Res 69: 228-33, 1999]

The right form of B12

Nearly all multivitamins provide vitamin B12 in the form of cyanocobalamin. However, most of the B12 naturally circulating in the blood plasma is in the methyl form. This form of vitamin B12 may not be easily utilized or as effective as methylcobalamin. For example, in some cases of optic nerve disease due to the toxic effects of tobacco or alcohol, methylcobalamin, but not cyanocobalamin, resolves the problem. [Seminars in Ophthalmology 10: 195-202, 1995] Cyanocobalamin does not reduce homocysteine levels whereas methylcobalamin does. Methylcobalamin increases the body's level of SAMe (S-adenosylmethionine), often employed as a food supplement to overcome mental depression and inflammation.

Recent research reveals that vitamin B12 as cobalamin needs to be complexed with glutathione, a universal antioxidant produced within living cells, in order to offer optimal protection from Alzheimer's disease. [Neurology 58: 1395-99, 2002] The provision of glutathione, or other sulfur-containing nutrients that boost glutathione such as alpha lipoic acid, with vitamin B12 is desirable in multivitamins.

< 52 >

Furthermore, the Food & Drug Administration has recently begun to fortify foods with folic acid, another B vitamin. [J Am Medical Assn 271: 1687-89, 1994] Folic acid can mask or hide a vitamin B12 deficiency. There is a strong likelihood that more undetected cases of pernicious anemia will occur in the adult population. [Environmental Nutrition 21: 6, 1998] If multivitamins provide at least 300 mcg of vitamin B12 the hidden plague of pernicious anemia would be minimized.

How do you know if you are deficient in vitamin B12? Blood tests may be helpful, but even persons in the normal range often notice beneficial changes in their health and energy levels when taking high-dose vitamin B12 supplements.

Recommended Daily Allowance Vitamin B12	Typical daily intake from foods	Amount needed for adults to avoid signs of deficiency
2.4 mcg	5.0 mcg	300-1000 mcg
Adults over age 50 advised to obtain vitamin B12 from fortified foods or supplements due to poor absorption	Common form of vitamin B12 in food supplements: cyanocobalamin	Predominant form of vitamin B12 in the blood circulation: methylcobalamin

Bottom line: Make sure your vitamin pill is designed to keep up with the latest science. Optimal levels of nutrients should be provided to deliver all of the health benefits widely reported in clinical studies. Adults who are middle-aged and older should consume a minimum of 300 mcg of supplementary vitamin B12, preferably as highly absorbable methylcobalamin.

< 53 >

Forget to take your vitamins?
Multivitamins may help prevent forgetfulness

Did you forget to take your vitamins today? There may be a reason why? The brain can store a quadrillion bits of information during a lifetime. From the age of 20 onward, about 50,000 nerve cells are lost daily, mainly from the brain cortex. The decline in memory, in particular short-term memory, begins as early as age 25. In 1991 researchers tested the ability of adults to learn and remember written information. From age 25 to age 49 there is a 21 percent decline in memory; by age 70-79 there is a 43 percent memory decline. [Archives Clinical Neuropsychology 6: 287-300, 1991]

B vitamins improve memory

Just look at the rate of memory decline with advancing age.

Ability to remember names one hour after introduction (Compared to 25-year olds)
Memory declines by 35 percent among 40-49 year olds
Memory declines by 47 percent among 50-59 year olds
Memory declines by 62 percent among 60-69 year olds
Memory declines by 74 percent among 70-79 year olds
Developmental Neuropsychology 9: 103-13, 1993

The good news is that there is a breakthrough in memory enhancement and brain cell preservation. We now know what the *"memory molecule"* is – it's called acetycholine, one of many chemical carriers of nerve impulses. A characteristic of senility is the reduced ability of the brain to produce acetycholine. With advancing age, the acetycholine production in brain cells drops by 70-80 percent.

How do we get more acetycholine for the brain? The family of B vitamins is involved in the manufacture of the memory molecule (acetycholine). Pantothenic acid, vitamin B5, promotes the production of acetycholine. [British Journal Pharmacology 95: 77-82, 1988] Vitamin B1 (thiamin)

< 54 >

is also involved in the release of acetycholine at the gaps (synapses) between nerve cells. High-dose vitamin B1 can defeat memory loss caused by a drug that induces amnesia. [Annals Neurology 34: 724-26, 1993] In Britain, young adult females who consumed 50 milligrams of vitamin B1 daily for two months produced reports of being *"more clearheaded, composed and energetic, "*but had no influence upon memory. [Psychopharmacology 129: 66-71, 1997] Vitamin B1 also helps to control sugar (glucose) levels, which is important in the release of acetycholine. [Proceedings Nutrition Society 58: 427-33, 1999]

Another link between memory impairment/brain aging and B vitamins is homocysteine. This is an undesirable blood protein that is linked with cardiovascular and brain disease. Homocysteine levels are reduced with folic acid, vitamin B12 and to a lesser extent by vitamin B6. One study shows that only those senior adults with very low vitamin B12 and folic acid levels experience memory impairment. [Psychology Aging 11: 487-96, 1996] In a more recent study, Swedish researchers found that folic acid is even more important than vitamin B12 in memory tests conducted among very old adults (age 90-101 years). [Biological Psychiatry 45: 1472-80, 1999] Among males age 54-81, high homocysteine levels have been linked with low vitamin B6 and B12 levels and poor performance on mental recognition tests. [American Journal Clinical Nutrition 63: 306-14, 1996] Vitamin B6 also plays a role in memory. Provision of 20 milligrams of vitamin B6 among men between the ages of 70-79 years of age helped to improve memory in a study conducted in the Netherlands. [Psychopharmacology 109: 489-96, 1992]

Antioxidants rescue brain neurons

Antioxidants, such as vitamin C, vitamin E and glutathione, serve as anti-rusting agents, protecting brain cells from premature aging and disease. In mice, the administration of high-dose vitamin C completely prevented drug-induced amnesia. [Neurobiology Learning Memory 64: 119-24, 1995] In Switzerland, adults age 65-94 years of age, higher circulating vitamin C and beta carotene levels are correlated with improved memory and vocabulary. [Journal American Geriatric Society

< 55 >

45: 718-24, 1997] In an elderly population of US adults, the ability to recall events or facts was diminished with low circulating levels of vitamin E. [American Journal Epidemiology 150: 37-44, 1999]

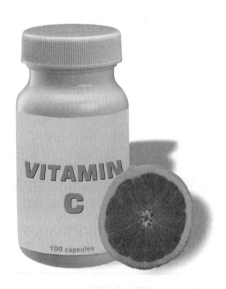

Get More Vitamin C
The false idea that americans are wasting their money
on high doses of vitamin C

How much vitamin C?		
To prevent scurvy	30 mg	Half an orange
Recommended intake	90 mg	1 1/2 oranges
Average dietary consumption	110 mg	Almost 2 oranges
To prevent cataracts	300-2000 mg	5-33 oranges
To control blood pressure	500 mg	8 oranges
To replace vitamin C in smokers (pack a day habit)	500 mg	8 oranges

Does mega-dose vitamin C produce expensive urine?

Americans purchase vitamin C more so than any other food supplement. <u>A recent survey reveals that better than 7 in 10 Americans purchase vitamin C supplements from time to time.</u> [Natural Marketing

< 56 >

Institute 2002] Over the years various dubious studies, which for some unexplained reason received widespread attention in the news media, have attempted to shake American consumers away from taking high-dose vitamin C.

There has been a long-standing myth that high-dose vitamin C is worthless. There is a false argument that excessive levels of vitamin C in vitamin pills are washed away in the urine and that Americans waste their money when buying mega-dose vitamins. This falsehood is based upon studies of levels of nutrients in the blood circulation, not tissue levels of nutrients. Many researchers indicate it is tissue levels of nutrients that count, not the amount circulating in the blood stream. For example, the adrenal glands and the eyes have much higher levels of vitamin C than the blood stream. Vitamin C concentration in the brain exceeds that of the blood by 10-fold. [Journal Clinical Investigation 100: 2842, 1997]

> **High-dose vitamin C is not just washed away in the urine**

A 1991 study, conducted at the USDA Human Nutrition Research Center on Aging at Tufts University, found that there were *"striking differences"* in ocular levels of vitamin C among older adults who consume 148 mg of vitamin C from their daily diet (which is 2.5 times the old 60 mg RDA and 1.6 times the current 90 mg recommendation) compared to adults who took 2000 mg daily from supplements. The level of vitamin C in the focusing lens and aqueous fluid of the eye increased by 22-32 percent with consumption of 2000 mg of daily vitamin C supplementation, which affords protection against cataracts. Thus the idea that vitamin C levels reach a saturation point at about 240 mg in the blood serum, and that additional vitamin C is worthless and only washes out in the urine, is dispelled by this research. [Current Eye Research 8: 751-59, 1991] This is the same level of vitamin C health authorities now consider *"risky."* [NAS press release April 10, 2000] Furthermore, antagonists use false reasoning since they never indict excessive levels of prescription drugs as causing *"expensive urine."*

< 57 >

It is a fact that the water-soluble vitamins are not retained or stored within the body and thus require greater intake. The fact that nutrients are washed away in the urine is more evidence for everyday replacement.

Common Myths About Vitamin C Supplements	
Myth	Truth
Myth: Once the saturation point is reached for vitamin C in the blood circulation the remaining excess is excreted in the urine. Thus mega-dose vitamin C is worthless.	Tissue levels of vitamin C are more important than blood levels. Vitamin C levels in the eyes and brain rise with intake of mega-dose vitamin C. Tissue levels of vitamin C exceed blood levels by many times. [Current Eye Research 8: 751-59, 1991; Journal Clinical Investigation 100: 2842, 1997]
Myth: Vitamin C pills cause kidney stones.	Numerous studies do not confirm that unfounded suspicion that vitamin C causes kidney stones. [J Urology 155: 1847-51, 1996; Ann Nutrition Met 41: 269-82, 1997; J Am Soc Neph 10: 840-45, 1999; Journal Urology 151: 834-37, 1994]
Myth: Vitamin C damages DNA	Five human studies show up to 10,000 milligrams of supplement vitamin C does not damage DNA. [Science 293:1993-5, 2001]
Myth: High-dose (500 mg) of vitamin C thickens neck (carotid) arteries. [Presentation, American Heart Assn, March 2000]	High-dose vitamin C builds collagen and thickens artery walls which can mistakenly be construed to mean blood vessels are narrowing.

How did the 90 mg recommended daily dose come about?

The new recommendations call for 90 mg for vitamin C for healthy adults, up from 60 mg per day under the previous standard. Yet health authorities keep preaching five servings of fresh fruits and vegetables, which supplies more than 200 mg of vitamin C. [Am J Clin Nut 62:

< 58 >

1347-56S, 1995] These two figures don't correlate. Just months before the 90 mg vitamin C recommendation was issued, various government scientists were calling for 120-200 mg per day in published reports. [Proc Natl Acad Sci 93: 3704-09, 1996; Nutrition Reviews 57: 222-24, 1999; Am J Clin Nut 69: 1086-1107, 1999] One researcher at the Massachusetts Institute of Technology, Laboratory of Human Nutrition, using a technique called saturation kinetics, suggested that even the 200 mg level was not adequate to meet individual vitamin C needs by as much as 2-3 fold. [Proc Natl Acad Sci 93: 14344, 48, 1996]

While the Food & Nutrition Board suggested adding another 35 mg of vitamin C for smokers (125 mg total), researchers at the Medical College of Wisconsin found that it takes 200 mg of vitamin C before smokers achieve the same serum levels of ascorbic acid as non-smokers. [Am J Clin Nut 53: 1466-70, 1991] Other investigators have called for 200 mg daily consumption of vitamin C for smokers. [Ann NY Acad Sci 686: 335-46, 1993] Swedish investigators demonstrated that a single 2000 mg dose of vitamin C can completely abolish the typical reduction in blood circulation that occurs while smoking a cigarette. A 1000 mg dose had no effect. [Microvascular Res 58: 305-11, 1999]

What happened to these recommendations? Health authorities conveniently stopped short of recommending levels of vitamin C that would require supplementation. The Academy of Sciences set the tolerable upper limit at 2000 mg, but a recent review indicated doses of vitamin C up to 4000 mg are well tolerated. [Nut Rev 57: 71-77, 1999] Eight placebo-controlled, double-blind studies and six non-placebo clinical trials in which up to 10,000 mg of vitamin C was consumed daily for up to 3 years confirm the safety of vitamin C in high doses. [J Am Coll Nut 14: 124-36, 1995] Yet the news headlines read *"huge doses considered risky."*

Furthermore, a member of the panel that established the 90 mg daily dose for vitamin C says there is *"no evidence that proves antioxidant supplements will help people live longer."* [Whole Foods Magazine, August 2000] Really? There was a UCLA study which showed that greater

< 59 >

than 300 mg of daily vitamin C increases the male life span by six years, a report that was widely reported in Newsweek and other periodicals. [Epidemiology 3: 194-202, 1992] A recent study confirms that finding. [Epidemiology 11: 440-45, 2000]

Additionally, one study shows that about 294 mg of vitamin C significantly decreases the risk of cataracts compared to 77 mg per day (about the level set by the Academy of Sciences). [Clin Chem 39: 1305, 1993] To get that much vitamin C a person would have to consume five oranges per day. Daily consumption of vitamin C supplements for 10 years or more results in a 77-83 percent reduction in the prevalence of cataracts. [Am J Clin Nut 66: 911-16, 1997]

Vitamin C and Blood Pressure

Recently researchers have discovered that a common cause of high blood pressure is the inability of blood vessels to widen (dilate) as the heart rate increases. Upon increased physical **500 mg vitamin C reduces blood pressure** demand the adrenal glands secrete a hormone (acetycholine) that widens the blood vessels. Also, a temporary gas called nitric oxide is released by cells lining the inside of blood vessels which causes dilation. But cholesterol plaques, smoking and the failure to produce nitric oxide will elevate blood pressure beyond normal limits. Mega-dose vitamin C restores the mechanism to control blood pressure by affecting all of the above factors. [Free Radical Biology Med 28: 1421-29, 2000] One study shows that 500 mg of supplemental vitamin C mildly reduces blood pressure (2.8 to 4.5 points) among middle-aged adults with hypertension. Doses greater than 500 mg had no effect. [Am J Therapy 9: 289-93, 2002]

< 60 >

Blood pressure is the measurement
of force applied to artery walls

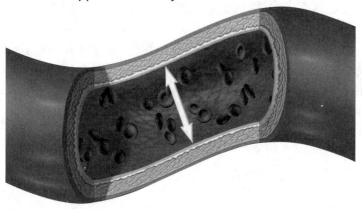

✿A.D.A.M.

500 milligrams of supplemental vitamin C has been shown to help
the blood vessels dilate (widen) in response to stress and thus help
maintain healthy blood pressure.

How much vitamin C?

The dosage of vitamin C requires some study by informed consumers.
How much vitamin C should adults consume? A lot more than many
people think. What's needed to prevent symptoms of scurvy (bleeding
gums, easy skin bruising, eye hemorrhages, anemia, fatigue)? Only
about 30 milligrams say researchers. Most vitamin supplements provide
at least 60 mg of vitamin C, and updated versions will provide 90 mg
since new guidelines call for 75 mg for females and 90 mg for males, and
a bit more for smokers. The average daily consumption of vitamin C
in the US is about 109 mg. A survey of vitamin C intake from dietary
sources reveals 18 percent had low vitamin C intake and 24 percent had
marginally low intakes. The remaining 58 percent were considered to
have adequate intake levels, that is, 60 milligrams per day (one orange a
day). [Eur J Clin Nut 54: 573, 2000] However, the adequate amount of
vitamin C is determined by the absence of scurvy, which would be the
minimal amount.

< 61 >

Researchers have attempted to determine the optimal amount of vitamin C consumption by measuring markers of oxidation (rusting) in blood samples. Young volunteers were given increasing amounts of supplemental vitamin C, starting with 75 mg, then every two weeks increasing intake to 250 mg, 500 mg, 1000 mg and finally 2000 mg. Markers of oxidation continued to drop up to about 1000 mg per day and there was no significant further benefit exhibited beyond that dose. [J Am College Nut, Vol. 20, No. 6, 2001] So is 1000 mg per day the optimal amount for human daily intake? The answer is no.

Mutant humans: vitamin C starved

Humans once produced vitamin C in their own bodies. Back in human history, prior to a universal genetic mutation, vitamin C was a hormone produced in the human liver. In reality, all humans are hopelessly vitamin C deficient because our early ancestors produced their own vitamin C naturally by the enzymatic conversion in the liver of circulating blood sugars to ascorbic acid. Most animals except for some species of fruit bats, fish, guinea pigs and some primates, produce their own vitamin C.

Humans have a defective gene in their liver which no longer produces the fourth enzyme (gulonolactone oxidase) required to produce vitamin C. [Am J Med 26: 740-48, 1959] Animals that produce vitamin C live 8-12 times beyond their age of physical maturation. Humans mature physically at about age 18 and live only 2.0-3.5 times beyond this. Reinstallation of the gene for the missing enzyme would extend the human life span to hundreds of years. Obviously, at some time in the past humans lived a lot longer than they do now. Maybe there is an element of truth to those Bible stories about Adam and Noah and Methuselah living so long.

Humans no longer make their own vitamin C as do animals

Animals produce about 60 milligrams of vitamin C per kilogram (2.2 pounds) of body weight, or for a 150 pound human would need about

< 62 >

4000 milligrams to reach the level once produced naturally within the body. Think of what the human body would be like with continual production of vitamin C. Since increased stress hormones signal for the release of stored sugars into the blood circulation, under stress humans would produce more vitamin C. Humans would no longer be vulnerable to the physical consequences of stress-related disease. There would be no diabetes since sugar would convert to ascorbic acid. Humans would renew their tissues more readily since collagen production would be elevated. Joints wouldn't wear out. Blood vessels wouldn't weaken with advancing age. Cataracts, kidney stones and other maladies would be a thing of the past. Scientists estimate humans need about 2000-4000 mg of vitamin C, taken at intervals through the day, to approximate what the human body once produced when vitamin C was a hormone, not a vitamin. [Medical Hypotheses 5: 711-21, 1979]

Humans Lost Their Ability to Produce Vitamin C Long Ago Most Animals Produce Their Own Vitamin C by the Enzymatic Conversion of Blood Sugar to Ascorbic Acid* *Except for some species of guinea pigs, fruit bats, fish and primates Daily Production of Vitamin C in Humans and Animals		
Humans and Animals	Milligrams of vitamin C produced per kilogram (2.2 pounds) of body weight/per day	If humans were the same weight as these animals, how much vitamin C would humans produce per day? (in milligrams)
Snake	10	700
Tortoise	7	490
Mouse	275	19,250
Rabbit	226	15,820
Goat	190	13,300
Rat	150	10,500
Dog	40	2800
Cat	40	2800
Humans	0	—
* Chart provided courtesy of Rusty Hoge of cforyourself.com. Cforyourself is the Internet's leading website about the nutritional benefits of vitamin C for optimum health. Visit cforyourself.com.		

< 63 >

Why humans are vulnerable to stress

But even this amount of vitamin C may not be enough. Stress triggers production of adrenal hormones which signals stored sugars and fats to be released into the blood circulation. Upon passage through the liver, these sugars would then be converted into vitamin C via an enzymatic process. This is how synthetic vitamin C is produced today, from corn syrup and enzymes. In animals that produce their own vitamin C, the more stress they experience the more vitamin C their bodies produce. An animal about the size of a human, such as a 160-pound mountain goat, produces about 13,000 milligrams of vitamin C per day and more under stress. [Med Hypotheses 5: 711, 1979] Vitamin C is an anti-stress vitamin and requirements vary depending upon the level of physical or emotional stress. A fixed intake level for vitamin C does not take into consideration varying levels of stress.

Sunshine in a bottle: get more vitamin D

Probably the first thing you will hear about vitamin D is that it is toxic in high doses. Virtually every nutrition textbook warns of a buildup of this fat-soluble vitamin in the liver with high-dose supplementation as well as calcium overload. This hardly seems plausible. For one thing, only small amounts, micrograms of this vitamin, are being produced in the skin by exposure to sunlight. Total body exposure to unfiltered sunlight in a southern latitude in the summer for one hour will produce about 10,000 International Units (IU) of vitamin D, which is only 250 micrograms (1/4th of 1 milligram). That is the equivalent of 100 glasses of fortified milk or 25 conventional vitamin pills. Men living in the Midwest exposed to summer sun are estimated to produce 2800 IU of vitamin D. [J Clin Endocrinology Metab 87: 4952, 2002] There are simply no reported cases of vitamin D toxicity due to sun poisoning. Obviously the body can handle a lot more vitamin D than previously thought. Reinhold Vieth PhD, world expert on vitamin D, says *"pharmacists almost always warn patients against taking the highest dose of vitamin D available over the counter (1000 IU, 25 mcg). They are warning patients against taking*

< 64 >

the very dose that adults need to ensure that vitamin D concentration exceed insufficiency." [Am J Clin Nut 74: 862-67, 2001]

A daily 5000 IU supplement (1250 mcg per day) has been taken for 8 weeks by males with no calcium overload. [J Assoc Physicians India 32: 185-86, 1984] The Merck Manual says toxic effects of vitamin D can occur in adults, but 100,000 IU (2500 mcg) is required for several months. [Merck Manual Diagnosis Therapy, Section 1, Chp. 3] All known cases of toxicity involve doses

> **The world death rate rises in winter when vitamin D levels are low**

exceeding 40,000 IU (1000 mcg) per day for extended periods of time. A recent study showed that 4000 IU per day is non toxic. [Am J Clin Nut 69: 842-56, 1999] The new safe upper limit is 2000 IU per day.

How much vitamin D to prevent bone loss?

Just 200 IU (5 mcg) of vitamin D is needed to prevent bone softening in the absence of sunlight, but more is needed to help prevent loss of bone density (osteoporosis) and secondary hyperparathyroidism. The new Daily Reference Intake level for vitamin D is a paltry 200 IU. For comparison, a teaspoon of cod liver oil provides 400 IU (10 micrograms) of vitamin D.

Except for people living near the equator, 800 to 3000 IU vitamin D intake is required to reduce fracture risk in older adults, since vitamin D regulates the absorption of calcium required for bone mineralization. [N Eng J Med 327: 1637, 1992; 337: 670, 1997] Vitamin D also increases magnesium absorption. [Mag Res 8: 19, 1995] To optimize health the leading vitamin D researcher in the world suggests supplementation exceeding 800 IU per day. Other researchers also recommend at least 800 IU of vitamin D both to improve calcification of bones and maintain muscle function in order to reduce hip fractures in frail elderly adults. [Osteoporosis 13: 187-94, 2002] Dark-skinned individuals living in northern latitudes (Seattle, Chicago, Detroit, Boston, Alaska) may need

< 65 >

to consume high-dose vitamin D supplements to maintain bone density and a healthy immune system.

Other health benefits of vitamin D

Vitamin D plays a role in diseases that occur more frequently in geographical areas where there is cloud cover for much of the year and decreased natural vitamin D production. The colon, breast and prostate cancer belt runs in Northern latitudes. Autoimmune disorders such as multiple sclerosis, arthritis and diabetes also correlated with these regions. [Proc Soc Exp Biol Med 223: 230-33, 2000] Multiple sclerosis requires more than genetic predisposition, it requires an environmental trigger such as the lack of vitamin D. [Proc Nut Soc 59: 531-35, 2000] Blood pressure rises at increasing distances from the equator and also rises in winter months and among people with dark skin pigmentation who make less vitamin D upon skin exposure to the sun. [Hypertension 30: 150-56, 1997]

The highest rates of colon, breast and prostate cancer correlate geographically with areas of cloud cover where natural vitamin D production is low in humans. Low dietary intake of vitamin D is linked with osteoarthritis of the knee. [Annals Int Med 125: 353, 1996] Vitamin D deficiency can also lead to muscle weakness and limb pain. [J Am Geriatric Soc 43: 833, 1995]

Benefits of vitamin D supplementation include prevention of osteoporosis, some cancers, multiple sclerosis, arthritis, muscle weakness, high blood pressure and the enhancement of the immune system. There is no toxicity from this amount of supplemental vitamin D. [Am J Clin Nut 69: 842-56, 1999]

How many are deficient in vitamin D?

Homebound Americans have been found to consume about 517 IU per day of vitamin D from the diet and exhibit very low circulating vitamin

< 66 >

D levels, only about 40 percent of what is needed. Incidental exposure of 5 percent of the skin surface to sunlight would end up with about half the population short of this vitamin.

Among 290 consecutive patients admitted to a medical ward in Massachusetts, 57 percent were considered to be vitamin D deficient including 43 percent of the patients with dietary intake above the Recommended Daily Allowance. [N Eng J Med 338: 777-83, 1998] A third of men living in Canada have been found to be deficient in vitamin D. [Can Med Assn J 166: 1541, 2002] One study showed that 43 percent of hospitalized patients consumed foods that exceeded the Recommended Daily Allowance for Vitamin D but were still vitamin-D deficient! [New Eng J Med 338: 777, 1998]

Bottom line: Multivitamins should provide adults with a minimum of 800 IU (20 mcg), the amount shown to reduce bone fractures, from natural-source vitamin D3 (not the synthetic vitamin D2 used to fortify milk). Adults living in Northern latitudes may require 1000 IU or more per day. [Can Med Assn J 166: 1541, 2002] Extra vitamin D should be provided in bone/mineral formulas and 2000 to 4000 IU per day can be taken safely in addition to 800 IU in multivitamins. This is ten times lower than the potential toxic level, which is 40,000 IU (1000 mcg). The safe upper limits on vitamin D need to be re-thought.

< 67 >

Some of the Benefits of Taking a Well-Designed Multivitamin

- Reduced infections, colds, flu, sickdays

- Convenience; reduces number of supplements taken daily

- Improves mental function, short-term working memory

- Saves money. Individual supplements are very costly.

- Covers 95%+ of the nutritional needs. Minmizes any nutritional shortages.

- Improves ability to handle physical and emotional stress

- Long-term users, reduces risk of cataracts and other eye disease

- Improves response to vaccinations

< 68 >

- Minimizes damage caused by homocysteine

- Provides levels of nutrients that the best diet cannot provide

- Reduces risk of chronic disease; slows aging

< 69 >

Vitamin Truth #5
The Power of Nutrient
Combinations

Nutrients have working companions. Antioxidant supplements are more powerful when water-soluble (watery) and fat-soluble (fatty) antioxidants are combined. [Lipids 31: 47-50, 1996] There are remote compartments within living cells and tissues that can easily be penetrated by watery or fatty nutrients, but not both.

The value of combined nutrients becomes apparent upon review of scientific studies. Vitamin B6 improves the potency of magnesium and selenium. [J Nutrition Science Vitaminology 37: 509-16, 1991] Vitamin C levels remain higher for longer periods of time when accompanied by bioflavonoids. Selenium and vitamin E work together to produce an important antioxidant enzyme (glutathione peroxidase). Vitamin D helps to maintain adequate levels of calcium. [Journal American Dietetic Assn 98: 699-706, 1998] So multiple nutrients, provided in a well-designed multivitamin, have advantages over singular food supplements or poorly-designed multivitamins with few ingredients.

Most nutritional research involves the study of a single nutrient. As consumers learn about the health benefits of specific nutrients, they are inclined to purchase these products. In recent years there has been a flood of information about nutritional supplements, which tends to overwhelm consumers. Some vitamin buyers will limit their consumption to one or two supplements. Others will opt for a multivitamin, to "cover the bases" so to speak. This is important since nutrients work together in the body.

Only recently have researchers begun to study multiple antioxidants and other nutrients. Nutrients work synergistically in the human body, that is, their sum works better than any singular nutrient. Recently healthy middle-aged males were given supplements providing vitamin

< 70 >

C, vitamin E and beta carotene. The circulating levels of vitamin E were much higher when vitamin E was taken with the other antioxidants than when taken alone. [J Am College Nutrition 15: 159-61, 1996] US Department of Agriculture researchers at Tufts University conducted a study among adults over age 60. When more than 220 mg of vitamin C was consumed, blood plasma levels of vitamin E were 18 percent higher. Vitamin C also raised beta carotene levels. [Am J Clinical Nutrition 62: 1228-33, 1995]

In an animal study, a cocktail of nine antioxidants (which included vitamin E, vitamin C, selenium, beta carotene, N acetyl cysteine, coenzyme Q10 and bioflavonoids) provided more protection against oxidation than vitamin E and selenium only. [Free Radical Biology & Medicine 20: 165-73, 1996] Researchers at the State University of New York recently reported when vitamin E is combined with bioflavonoids such as quercetin, the antioxidant protection in the eye is enhanced. [Ophthalmic Research 28: 184-92, 1996] Harvard researchers used a mixture of antioxidants (beta carotene, vitamin E, glutathione and vitamin C) and found they reduced the size and quantity of tumors in animals while vitamin C alone actually increased tumors. [Nutrition & Cancer 20: 145-51, 1993]

A compelling animal study conducted by Harvard researchers shows how antioxidants work synergistically. Groups of five animals were given a tumor-promoting chemical and various antioxidants. View the results of the study in the chart below.

Antioxidants - In animals with tumors	No. of tumors
Control group/no antioxidants	17
Vitamin C	15
Beta carotene	7
Vitamin E	7
Glutathione	6
Mixture of all antioxidants above	2
Source: Nutrition & Cancer 20: 145-51, 1993	

< 71 >

In a test tube study, researchers at the University of Colorado also found that low-dose vitamin C actually stimulates growth of tumor cells, but at a high concentration, inhibits tumor growth. Vitamin C, beta carotene, vitamin A and vitamin E combined were the most effective at inhibiting tumors. The researchers concluded that, *"the use of multiple antioxidant vitamins is essential for a maximal reduction in cancer incidence among a high-risk population. The use of one or two vitamins may be ineffective or even harmful."* [Nutrition & Cancer 26: 11-19, 1996]

Homocysteine is an undesirable blood protein whose levels are particularly high among individuals who do not eat fresh vegetables. When homocysteine levels are intentionally elevated in small animals their memory is impaired whereas if the animals are pre-treated with very high doses of vitamins E and C, memory loss is prevented. [Metab Brain Disease 17: 211-17, 2002]

A significant percentage of adults only supplement their diet with vitamin C or vitamin E. They are likely missing the many health benefits provided by a well-designed multivitamin.

Air, moisture and light combine to oxidize the bumper of your car. In time the bumper will rust away. This destructive process is called oxidation. To explain this another way, remove the antioxidant coating from an apple by peeling away its skin and exposing the insides of the apple to the air. It will spoil quickly. Pour lemon juice, which contains antioxidants, on the exposed apple and it will delay spoilage.

All living cells must breathe oxygen. A by-product of cellular respiration is the production of a small number of toxic oxygen molecules called *"free radicals."* These are atoms that are missing an electron. So they go searching to steal electrons from nearby atoms and in doing so, destroy cells and tissues. Antioxidants stop the damaging free radical oxygen molecules. So as long as antioxidants, the *"rust removers"* of living cells, are abundant, oxidation will not destroy tissues and promote disease. But scientists estimate that the genetic material (DNA) inside living cells in the human body is being hit by 10,000 *"free radical"* bullets each day.

< 72 >

An antioxidant-rich diet and food supplements are likely to be needed to protect our genes.

THE ANTIOXIDANT TREE©		
RUSTING AGENTS		
Singlet Oxygen	Hydroxyl Radical Mainly iron induced	Superoxide Radical
ANTI-RUSTING AGENTS (antioxidants)		
Catalase (zinc, copper, manganese)	Glutathione (sulfur)	Superoxide Dismutase (zinc, copper, manganese)
Vitamin A	Vitamin C	Vitamin E Tocopherols, Tocotrienols
Carotenoids Beta carotene Lutein/ zeaxanthin Lycopene	Bioflavonoids	Coenzyme Q10

The human body has an elaborate antioxidant system to protect itself. The system, which I call *"The Antioxidant Tree,"* can be likened to a team of football players on defense. If you recall, a defensive team has some big lineman who are the front line against the opponent, backed up by linebackers and then by safety men. The antioxidant team in your body works in a similar fashion.

The first line of antioxidant defense are antioxidant enzymes which are naturally produced inside your body. There are three: glutathione, superoxide dismutase (SOD), and catalase.

The linebackers or second line of defense are vitamins A, C and E.

The third line of defense are the carotenoids, the bioflavonoids, and coenzyme Q10.

< 73 >

Each of these antioxidants can become oxidized themselves. Fortunately, other antioxidants come along and donate electrons to re-activate them. So antioxidants exist in two forms, their active (reduced) or oxidized form. Antioxidants whirl through living tissues, re-activating each other. Vitamins A, C and E protect each other in a circular fashion. Vitamin A regenerates vitamin C, vitamin C regenerates vitamin E, and vitamin E regenerates vitamin A.

The antioxidant system has other backup systems. For instance, beta carotene converts to vitamin A in the liver, so it is a backup to vitamin A. Bioflavonoids enhance and prolong the antioxidant action of vitamin C and coenzyme Q10 works in place of vitamin E when vitamin E levels are low.

Multivitamins should be formulated the way nature has arranged the antioxidant defense force, in an *"Antioxidant Tree."* If any portion of this antioxidant defense force is missing, a health problem may result.

Without having an array of antioxidants to protect them, living tissues perish. Just like a football team that may line up without all its players on the field, if there is a deficiency of just one antioxidant the opponent will find this weakness and capitalize on it.

Look at the section in this book on homocysteine, a toxic protein that circulates in the blood and destroys blood vessels, nervous tissues and various other organs. It takes a combination of nutrients to effectively reduce homocysteine, particularly folic acid and vitamin B12.

Have you noticed that I continually use the word *"supplement?"* It is a very careful choice of words. Never forget that vitamin pills are a supplement to a healthy diet, not a replacement for it. Foods and supplements are mutually exclusive.

Nutritionists accurately advise the public to consume more plant foods, the five daily servings of fresh fruits and vegetables, to supply the variety of nutrients required for health. We know that the best-made pills can

< 74 >

never supply the hundreds of natural antioxidants and other nutrients found in plant foods. For example, there are over 200 carotenoid pigments found in plant foods in miniscule amounts. It would be impossible to provide them all in vitamin supplements. However, with so few adults consuming the five servings of plant foods daily, a well-designed multivitamin pill becomes a realistic barrier against premature aging and disease.

< 75 >

Vitamin Truth #6
Keep Taking Your Vitamins

Consumers often want instant benefits when taking multivitamins. They want more energy, vigor, faster thinking, better memory and recall, increased immunity and protection from disease. Oftentimes multivitamins, particularly well-designed brands, deliver on these promises. We age slowly. The progression of aging and age-related disease is synonymous. Studies now reveal, for the first time, that long-term vitamin users experience health benefits over those who only occasionally take supplements. For example, since cataracts usually progress slowly, diminishing the transparency of the human eye by about 1 percent per year, the anti-cataract properties of vitamin supplements only become apparent among long-term users of vitamin supplements. [Epidemiology 10: 679-84, 1999] Long-term vitamin C users have a 70-80 percent reduced risk for cataracts. [Am J Clin Nut 66: 911-16, 1997] Regular vitamin E supplement use, for 10 years or more, is associated with reduced risk of bladder cancer mortality. Regular use for shorter periods of time does not reduce risk. [Am J Epidemiology 156: 1002-10, 2002]

< 76 >

Vitamin Truth #7
Not Vitamins But "Rightamins"

Consumers read that their multivitamin provides vitamin E, selenium, beta carotene, and other essential nutrients. But is the type of vitamin E, selenium and beta carotene the same as used in research studies? In many instances, no. Different varieties of nutrients are often used that provide no health benefit whatsoever, often because they are cheaper.

Get the Right Form of Vitamin E

Preference of Human Tissues For Natural-source Vitamin E from Soy Over Synthetic Vitamin E Derived From Petroleum		
Tissue	**Preference ratio for natural over synthetic vitamin E**	**Reference**
Cholesterol	1-to-1	Arterioscler Thromb 13: 601, 1993
Liver	2-to1	Natl Research Council Canada
Blood serum	3-to-1	Am J Clin Nut 65: 785, 1997
Placenta	3.5-to-1	Am J Clin Nut 67: 459, 1998
Red blood cells	4-6-to-1	Journal Nutrition 121: 454, 1991
Brain	5.3-to-1	Natl Research Council Canada

The official position is that natural-source vitamin E (d-alpha tocopherol, also referred to as rrr-alpha tocopherol) derived from soy is only marginally better than synthetically produced vitamin E

< 77 >

(dl-alpha tocopherol, also called rrr-all-rac tocopherol) derived from petroleum. Obviously politics prevail over good science. Generally it is stated that natural-source vitamin E, milligram for milligram, is only about 36 percent more bioavailable than synthetic vitamin E, not enough to warrant paying a lot of extra money for the real McCoy. But that is on a dosage basis, not how the tissues prefer and store vitamin E. There is a large difference in the bioavailability (absorption) of synthetic vitamin E and the accumulation and usage of vitamin E by various tissues in the body. Fatty tissues which need to be protected from turning rancid, such as those found in the brain, prostate, breast and retina, exhibit a stronger affinity for natural-source vitamin E over synthetic vitamin E. Red blood cells, which have to be protected from destruction as they rapidly travel throughout the circulatory system, also have a stronger affinity for natural-source vitamin E over synthetic E. With physical exercise, more vitamin E is released from adipose (fatty tissues) into the blood circulation to protect the red blood cells.

Burton Graham, noted vitamin E researcher at the National Research Council of Canada, Ottawa, says *"Both forms of vitamin E are absorbed equally well through the gut, but for example, the liver clearly prefers the natural form, transferring it to lipoproteins to be transported through the blood for deposition into the tissues. The natural vitamin E is retained by a two-to-one ratio in the liver over the synthetic."* Burton has reported brain tissues prefer natural-source vitamin E 5.3 times more than synthetic E. Burton's research along with other studies suggests a far greater disparity between natural and synthetic vitamin E. In light of this evidence German researchers have challenged the often-stated figure that natural-source vitamin E is only 36 percent more biopotent than synthetic E, stating the real figure ought to be more like a 2-to-1 biopotency factor (or more) for natural over synthetic vitamin E. The researchers said: *"Because natural and synthetic vitamin E are not chemically identical and differ in plasma and tissue kinetics and metabolism, the current ratio of bioavailability (absorption) does not reflect the ratio of biopotency (accumulation in tissues)."* [Eur J Nutr 39:183-93, 2000]

< 78 >

In summary, you can use 89 or 94 octane gasoline in your automobile, and that would only make a small difference, but if you have an engine that prefers and runs 3 to 5 times better on 94 octane than 89 octane, it would certainly be worth the price differential.

Unless consumers are very informed, they don't know the difference of one kind of vitamin E from another. You may be taking 100 units of vitamin E, but it may not have enough antioxidant power to protect your body from disease. Many brands of vitamin E print their labels as *"vitamin E"* rather than designate the exact form of vitamin E. So consumers have no way of knowing which type of vitamin E is

Two families of vitamin E: tocotrienols and tococopherols

provided. Natural-source vitamin E is a bit more expensive, but not 3-5 times more expensive. Consumers are not getting their money's worth when purchasing synthetic vitamin E. Most consumers can't remember there is only one letter that indicates the difference from natural (d) and synthetic vitamin E (dl). Some manufacturers use a different scientific nomenclature for vitamin E, which further confuses consumers. Natural vitamin E can also be labeled as rrr-alpha tocopherol and synthetic as all-rac alpha tocopherol. A Gallup poll shows that vitamin E is consumed by 32 percent of American households and 65 percent think they are taking natural-source vitamin E when only 24 percent are actually doing so. [Supplement Industry Executive Oct. 2000]

Natural-source vitamin E (soy)	Synthetic vitamin E (petroleum source)
Label will read.... d-alpha tocopherol or rrr-alpha tocopherol	Label will read.... dl-alpha tocopherol or all-rac alpha tocopherol

In a recent study, 2000 units of daily synthetic vitamin E (dl-alpha tocopherol) delayed the onset of Alzheimer's disease by about six months. [New England Journal Medicine 336: 1216-22, 1997] If a person were

< 79 >

taking natural-source vitamin E they may need far less dosage to achieve the same benefit.

The dry powdered form of vitamin E (succinate) is more easily absorbed than the oily form (acetate). So look for the dry form. [Townsend Letter for Doctors, Jan 1993] In test-tube studies, the dry form of vitamin E has been shown to be more effective than the oily form. [Toxicology 128: 113-24, 1998]

Some confusion arises over whether mixed forms of vitamin E should be provided. Scientists use Greek letters to designate the different types of vitamin E (called tocopherols) --- alpha, beta, delta and gamma.

Originally, when vitamin E first became available as a food supplement, it was only provided in the mixed forms (alpha, beta, delta and gamma). But only the alpha form of vitamin E is stored in fatty tissues and maintained in the body and remains at sufficient levels in the body to provide antioxidant protection. [Am J Clinical Nutrition 27: 980, 1974; J Nutrition 131: 369S, 2001] It was only when 75-80 percent of the vitamin E was comprised of alpha tocopherol that cases of angina subsided. This was proven by Drs. Evan and Wilfred Shute of Canada, who performed the original work on vitamin E and heart disease. [Am J Clinical Nutrition 49: 517, 1989; Vitamin E Book, Wilfred Shute, Keats Publishing, 1975] But most vitamin E supplements solely provide alpha tocopherol with no accompanying forms of other tocopherols. Recent studies point to the need to provide a full array of vitamin E-like molecules in vitamin supplements. See the section concening nutrient balance later in this book which emphasizes the importance of mixed forms of vitamin E (tocopherols and tocotrienols).

< 80 >

Vitamin C: Get the Right Form of Vitamin C

Alkaline mineral ascorbates

The form of vitamin C once produced in the human body was a mineral-salt-vitamin, that is, what is called a mineral ascorbate. In animals that produce their own vitamin C, this vitamin is complexed with sodium, calcium, magnesium and other minerals. This alkaline form of vitamin C is desired since it is not acid and irritating to sensitive stomach lining as is ascorbic acid.

Vitamin C is incomplete without bioflavonoids

When vitamin C was first isolated from foods in the 1930s it was synthesized and used to treat cases of scurvy. But the symptoms of scurvy didn't disappear in all the patients until bioflavonoids were added to the synthetic vitamin C. In 1937, doctors in Copenhagen reported that a few scurvy patients did not improve even when given 3000 mg of synthetic vitamin C orally and 300 mg of vitamin C intravenously. Until bioflavonoids from lemons were consumed, the patients didn't improve. [The Lancet, pp. 1363-65, Dec. 11, 1937] In fact the title of their report was *"The inadequacy of synthetic ascorbic acid (vitamin C) as an antiscorbutic agent."* This fact is often overlooked. Essentially all of the vitamin C in vitamin pills is synthetic because it would be excessively expensive to extract it from plants. Thus bioflavonoids are needed to make synthetic vitamin C effective.

Bioflavonoids are plant pigments that accompany vitamin C in plant foods. Bioflavonoids help to sustain blood levels of vitamin C, like natural time-release agents. Bioflavonoids also help to improve the absorption of vitamin C. [American J Clinical Nutrition 48: 601-04, 1988] In one study, four hours after consumption, vitamin C levels were 68 percent higher among those individuals who took bioflavonoids with vitamin C than those who consumed vitamin C alone. [Am J Clinical Nutrition 48: 601-04, 1988] Combined together, vitamin C and

< 81 >

bioflavonoids tighten blood capillaries which typically become weak in cases of scurvy. One-hundred milligrams of bioflavonoids that contain red and purple pigments improve capillary closure nearly eight times better than bioflavonoids derived from citrus fruit. [The Pharmacology of Plant Phenolics, J.W. Fairbairn, ed., Academic Press, pp. 81-90, 1959]

Without bioflavonoids, vitamin C is an incomplete vitamin. Bioflavonoids are obtained from the rind of citrus fruits and the seeds and skin of berries and grapes (blueberry, huckleberry, bilberry, cranberry, pomegranate, grape seed, pine bark, quercetin, etc.) In a study comparing bioflavonoids from fruits, cranberry exhibited the highest total antioxidant activity followed by apple, red grape, strawberry, pineapple, banana, peach, lemon, orange, pear and grapefruit. [J Agric Food Chem 50: 7449-54, 2002]

Many brands of vitamin C indicate bioflavonoids are provided on their label. But the amount of bioflavonoids provided in vitamin pills is often paltry, not enough to strengthen weak capillaries. Researchers suggest bioflavonoids should be provided in a ratio of at least 70 percent of the total vitamin C. [Journal American Dietetic Assn. 94: 779-81, 1994] For example, if 100 mg of vitamin C were provided, there should at least be an accompanying 70 mg of bioflavonoids. Sadly, many multivitamins do not provide bioflavonoids at all.

Another reason why vitamin C should be accompanied by bioflavonoids is that vitamin C increases the absorption of iron from foods. Trouble is, iron buildup is a potential problem for adults who are middle aged and older. Bioflavonoids are iron-binding antioxidants and thus counter this problem. [Biology Trace Element Research 62: 135-53, 1998]

The claim that esterified vitamin C is beneficial is only a fleeting benefit. Esterified vitamin C may initially yield higher blood levels of this vitamin, but two hours after consumption there is little difference in blood levels of plain vitamin C and esterified vitamin C. [Journal Optimal Nutrition 2: 205, 1993] Consumers may be paying 3.3 to 4.2 times more for this

< 82 >

form of vitamin C which is not superior in retention or absorption to vitamin C with ample amounts of accompanying bioflavonoids. [Journal Am Dietetic Assn. 94: 779-81, 1994] It's better to purchase a brand of vitamin C that provides ample amounts of bioflavonoids than it is to purchase esterified vitamin C.

Added note: A potent bioflavonoid that most consumers are likely to be unfamiliar with is quercetin. This bioflavonoid is found naturally in small amounts in red apples (7 mg) and red onions (30 mg). The diet provides about 11 mg of quercetin per day. [European J Clinical Nutrition 50: 63-71, 1996] Quercetin is nature's antihistamine and inhibits the replication of the herpes family of viruses. [Antiviral Res 22: 327-31, 1993]

> **Vitamin C is incomplete without bioflavonoids**

Quercetin has about 12 times more antioxidant activity as vitamin E. It is an excellent companion to vitamin C. [Am J Clin Nut 67: 1210-18, 1998]

Not only is vitamin C a more potent and complete vitamin when it is combined with bioflavonoids, but nutritional scientists can re-engineer vitamin C for better penetration into tissues. Vitamin C is a water-soluble vitamin. Generally, vitamin C doesn't pass through fatty membranes that make up the outside of living cells, nor does it easily pass through barriers in the brain, eyes and spinal cord. But vitamin C can be re-engineered into a fatty vitamin (ascorbyl palmitate) so it can pass more easily through fatty membranes.

Bottom line: About 500 mg is an optimal amount of vitamin C for multivitamins, this amount having been shown to improve longevity, prevent cataracts and reduce hypertension. The alkaline mineral-ascorbate form of vitamin C is desirable. More vitamin C may be taken though the day to mimic what the human body once naturally produced and to continually replace this easily excreted water-soluble vitamin. Bioflavonoids should accompany vitamin C and equal 70 percent of the milligrams of vitamin C. Bioflavonoids are provided in citrus, grapes,

< 83 >

berries (cranberry, cherries, blueberry), milk thistle, green tea and onions (quercetin).

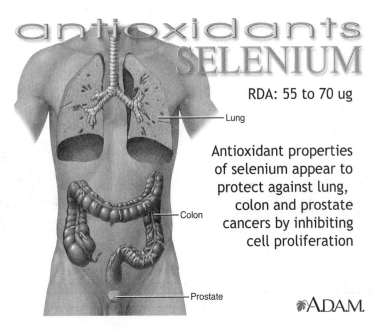

antioxidants
SELENIUM

RDA: 55 to 70 ug

Lung

Antioxidant properties of selenium appear to protect against lung, colon and prostate cancers by inhibiting cell proliferation

Colon

Prostate

🌿A.D.A.M.

Research studies reveal there are extra health benefits when humans consume 200 micrograms of organically-bound selenium from supplements.

The right kind of selenium

Selenium, a trace mineral, is another nutrient that consumers will want to scrutinize in the fine print found on multivitamin labels. There are two types of selenium provided in food supplements, inorganic (selenate, selenite) and organically-bound selenomethionine and selenium derived from Baker's yeast (SelenoExcel™) that is bound to an array of proteins (amino acids) as found naturally in foods. In recent years scientists have identified more

> **Use SelenoExcel, the same type of selenium successfully used in studies**

< 84 >

proteins bound to selenium. Supplemental selenium should be obtained in the same form it is found in plant foods.

The Third National Health and Nutrition Examination Survey found that 99 percent of subjects had adequate circulating levels of selenium. [Nutrition Clinical Care 5: 75, 2002] Yet when 200 milligrams of selenium was provided as an organically bound array of proteins (Seleno Excel™) significant reductions in the risk of cancer were found. [J Am Med Assoc 276: 1957-63, 1996] So maybe humans need more of this trace mineral than previously estimated. This study has now been extended a few more years and it continues to reveal a 50 percent drop in the relative risk for prostate cancer in males taking a selenium supplement. The protective effect is more pronounced among people with low intake levels of selenium. [Cancer Epid Biomarkers Prev 11: 630-39, 2002]

Selenium has other remarkable properties. <u>Mutations occurring in DNA of the influenza virus are of concern simply because they can create virulent strains that are quite lethal, such as the Spanish Flu that encircled the globe in 1918 and killed millions.</u> Selenium reduces the mutations in the influenza virus. [FASEB J 15:32, 2001] Selenium also protects against infection by the

Viruses can mutate without enough selenium

Coxsackie virus, a pathogen that can attack the heart muscle. [Biol Trace Elem Res 80: 23, 2001] In addition to iodine, selenium is needed for proper thyroid function. [Med Hypotheses 57: 480, 2001] Selenium has pervasive health benefits and researchers are beginning to describe this trace mineral as a true nutraceutical. [Current Opinion Clin Nutrition Metab Care 5: 659-63, 2002]

But many inexpensive brands of vitamins provide inorganic selenium as <u>sodium selenate</u> or <u>selenite</u>, which may <u>not</u> provide the same health benefits. The two prevalent organic forms of selenium in multivitamins are <u>selenomethionine</u>, which is selenium bound to one amino acid, methionine, and <u>SelenoExcel™ which is bound to any array of proteins</u>

< 85 >

as occurs naturally in foods. The full array of about 30 proteins bound to selenium in foods have only been identified in the past decade. [Public Health Nut 4: 593, 2001] Until more is known, it is advisable to consume the same array of protein-bound selenium molecules found only in a type of selenium supplement known as SelenoExcel™ since this was the form of supplement successfully used in the largest controlled study of selenium. By the way, organic selenium grown from yeast has no live yeast cells. It is not of concern to yeast-sensitive individuals.

In a clinical study, only organic selenium was recommended to reduce the risk of retinal disease, not sodium selenate or selenite. [Acta Ophthalmologica 76: 62-67, 1998]

Look for this kind of selenium in food supplements...	Not this kind......inorganic
Organically-bound selenium	**Inorganic selenium**
Selenomethionine	Selenate
SelenoExcel™ (preferred)	Selenite

Bottom line: Check the label on your daily vitamin pill to see if it provides the forms of nutrients that are highly absorbable and utilizable in human tissues. Look for d-alpha tocopherol for vitamin E (not dl-alpha tocopherol), organic selenium (SelenoExcel™) and absorbable forms of zinc (not zinc oxide nor magnesium oxide).

Alkaline mineral ascorbates (vitamin C complexed with minerals) are the preferred form of supplemental vitamin C. Vitamin C should be accompanied by bioflavonoids equaling at least 70 percent of the amount of vitamin C to prolong the action of vitamin C in the blood circulation.

< 86 >

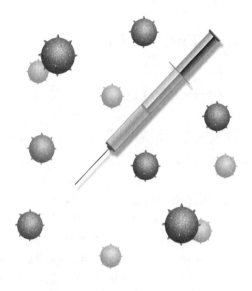

Antioxidant vitamins improve response to vaccines

Immunity and multivitamins

A significant percentage of senior adults cannot produce enough antibodies to adequately protect against disease. Successful response to the flu vaccine only occurs in 30 to 70 percent of senior adults. [Vaccine 12: 1185, 1994; 17: 82, 1999] Supplementation with zinc and selenium significantly improves the response rate to the flu vaccine among older adults. [Arch Intern Med 159: 748, 1999] Normally non-virulent viruses may convert to potentially harmful viruses when there is a shortage of vitamin E and selenium. [Proceed Nutrition Soc 58: 707, 1999] A 200 mg daily dose of vitamin E has been shown to improve the antibody response to tetanus, diphtheria and hepatitis B vaccines better than supplementation with lower (60 mg) or higher (800 mg) doses. [J Am Med Assn 277: 1380, 1997]

A daily multivitamin that provides around 20 milligrams of zinc, 100 micrograms of selenium and 200 IU of vitamin E appears to maintain immunity among older adults. [Clin Infectious Dis 33: 1892, 2001] A multivitamin providing vitamins C and E with beta carotene and trace minerals zinc and selenium has been shown to decrease the number of infections among senior adults. [Nutrition Reviews 55: 400, 1997]

< 87 >

Vitamin Truth #8
Learn What's Missing from Your Multivitamin Formula?

Scientists only began to isolate and identify vitamins as essential components of the human diet beginning in the 1930s. Discoveries and new findings have come out non-stop since then. There is a growing list of nutrients that some physiologists suggest be added to the list of essential nutrients. [Preventive Medicine 25: 46-47, 1996] Four of these are the trace mineral chromium, sulfur-bearing nutrients such as alpha lipoic acid, N-acetyl cysteine and taurine, an antioxidant called coenzyme Q10, and a yellow plant pigment called lutein. Unfortunately, few multivitamins today provide these four nutrients.

Chromium is a trace mineral that is essential for human health. Chromium is known for its ability to help control blood sugar levels, reduce resistance to insulin within living cells, lower cholesterol and reduce body fat. [Diabetic Medicine 13: 389-91, 1996; Nutrition Today 31: 226-33, 1996] A 200 mcg supplement of chromium has been shown to reduce *"bad"* LDL cholesterol and raise *"good"* HDL cholesterol. [Western J Medicine 152: 41-45, 1990] A study that employed 400 mcg supplemental chromium and 30 mg of zinc did not reduce blood sugar (hemoglobin A1c) in adult-onset diabetics, but the regimen did reduce markers of oxidation. [J Am College Nut 20: 212, 2001] However, greater amounts of chromium, more than 400 mcg, may be needed to produce sugar control in adult-onset diabetics. A number of studies confirm supplemental chromium may improve sugar control, insulin levels, cholesterol and hemoglobin A1c in adults with mild diabetes. [J Am College Nut 17: 548, 1998] Even childhood-onset diabetics may experience improvement in hemoglobin A1c levels when taking 600 mcg of chromium daily. [J Family Practice 46: 83, 1998] The National Academy of Sciences recommends Americans consume 50-200 mcg of chromium daily, but most Americans get less than 50 mcg daily from their diet.

< 88 >

No mention is made of sulfur in mineral supplements, but sulfur is as essential for life as any other mineral. (Please note, sulfur is not sulfa, which many people are allergic to.) Sulfur is an important nutrient because it is needed to make glutathione, the most important antioxidant in the body. Glutathione has been described as *"an essential cellular constituent, absolutely required for maintenance and survival"* of all biological systems. [Nature 224: 117-20, 1969] Another report says, *"Although glutathione is not considered an essential nutrient, under certain therapeutic conditions or in situations associated with environmental stress, a requirement for glutathione may become apparent."* [Glutathione: Metabolism and Physiological Functions, CRC Press, pp. 352-58, 1990]

Sulfur is absent from most vitamin pills

Americans consume somewhere between 25 and 125 mg of glutathione from plant foods in their daily diet. Glutathione is also provided in some multivitamin pills, though the liver will make up to 14,000 mg of glutathione per day if it is provided enough sulfur. [European J Clinical Nutrition 17: 408-14, 1987] Originally glutathione (glu-tah-thigh-on) was called philothione, derived from the Greek words philo (love) and thion (sulfur). Sulfur is provided in foods such as garlic, eggs, asparagus and onions. Taurine and methionine and N-acetyl cysteine are sulfur-bearing amino acids which are sometimes included in vitamin pills. Sulfur-bearing products such as DMSO and MSM are widely touted because of their ability to boost glutathione levels. The most easily absorbed source of sulfur is alpha lipoic acid which has been tested successfully as an antidote to diabetes, cataracts, and has been shown to help allay brain damage following a stroke. Better than 99 percent of alpha lipoic acid is absorbed compared to less than10 percent of N-acetyl cysteine [Eur J Clinical Pharmacology 34: 77-82, 1988], so it is regarded by Lester Packer, PhD, researcher at University of California at Berkeley, as the most potent glutathione booster that can be added to a vitamin pill. Glutathione boosters should be an essential component of every daily multivitamin because glutathione is required to sustain life. One-hundred milligrams or more of sulfur-bearing nutrients is a good starting point in a multivitamin formula. Studies have shown that glutathione

< 89 >

levels are low in states of disease and in one study only those adults who had high glutathione levels survived beyond age 79. Glutathione levels begin to decline with advancing age beginning at age 40 [J Lab Clinical Medicine 120: 720-25, 1992], so middle-aged adults and older adults should obtain some sources of sulfur in their daily vitamin pill.

Coenzyme Q10 is an antioxidant produced within the body. With advancing age less coenzyme Q10 is produced. Coenzyme Q10 is prescribed in doses exceeding 100 mg per day to help the heart beat stronger [J Orthomolecular Medicine 12: 4-10, 1997] and is also known for its ability to prevent cholesterol from hardening. [Proceedings Natl Academy Sciences 88: 1646-50, 1991] A 200 mg daily dose of CoQ10 has been shown to mildly reduce blood pressure among adult diabetics. [Eur J Clin Nut 56, 1137, 2002] Individuals who take cholesterol-lowering drugs may be at a greater risk to experience a shortage of coenzyme Q10. [Clin Invest 71: 137-139, 1993] While coenzyme Q10 is prohibitively expensive for most daily vitamin formulas, a low-dose may help to minimize age-related shortages.

< 90 >

Food Supplements That Help To Maintain Healthy Blood Pressure Levels			
Nutrient	Dosage/ day	Obtain from	References
Vitamin C	500 mg Moderate effect	Supplements	Am J Therapy 9: 289, 2002
Vitamin D	1000 IU+ Small effect	Sun exposure or supplements	Hypertension 30: 150, 1997; Am J Clin Nutr. 69: 842, 1999
Vitamin E	300 IU Small effect	Supplements	Am J Hypertension 13: 564, 2000
Vitamin B6	40-350 mg Ample effect Diabetics	Supplements	Molecular Cell Biochemistry, Volume 200, pages 155-62, October 1999; Arzneimittelfor Volume 45, 1271-73, 1995
Potassium (combine with low sodium intake)	500-1000 mg Ample effect	Foods (example: bananas 450 mg) Potassium is restricted in food supplements to 99 mg	Current Atheroscler Rep 2: 521, 2000; J Hum Hypertension 11: 7898, 1997
Coenzyme Q10	200 mg Ample effect Diabetics	Supplements	Eur J Clin Nut 56: 1137, 2002

Include Boron for Health

Boron is an overlooked mineral. Boron helps to normalize hormone levels in males and females and thus aids in maintaining bone mass as well as bone hardness.

Boron is important for maintaining hard bones and in maintaining hormone levels in males and females. Orthopedists have found that bones are much harder in areas where boron levels are high in the

< 91 >

water supply. In animals, boron improves the resistance of the long-leg bones (femur) to bending pressure. [Fund Applied Toxicol 35: 205, 1997] A daily 3 milligram boron supplement, the amount provided by diets high in fruits and vegetables, prevents loss of calcium and bone demineralization. [FASEB Journal 1: 394: 1987] Low boron intake may induce hyper-absorption of calcium. [British J Nut 69: 871-84, 1993]

Boron and hormones

The same amount of boron improves the blood serum concentration of estrogen in postmenopausal women. [Env Health Perspect 102: 59, 1994] Boron has been found to work in a similar fashion to hormone replacement therapy (estrogen) in preventing the loss of calcium from bone. [J Trace Elem Exp Med 3: 45-54, 1990]

Another study shows that a 3 mg boron supplement has been shown to reduce the urinary excretion of calcium and magnesium and markedly increased concentrations of estrogen and testosterone in women. [FASEB J 1: 394-97, 1987] The role of boron in normalizing hormone levels is of increased significance given that hormone replacement therapy has now been largely abandoned since estrogen replacement has not been found to prevent disease, and may actually increase health risks among postmenopausal women. [J Am Med Assn 288: 334, 2002; J Cardiovascular Risk 9: 309, 2002]

Boron helps maintain hormone levels

Because of boron's ability to modulate hormone levels, males who consume nearly 2 milligrams of boron from dietary sources, such as fruits and nuts, exhibit a 64 percent reduction in the risk for prostate cancer. The consumption of four servings of fruit and nuts per day would provide 3 to 6 milligrams of boron. [Science News 159: No. 15, 2001]

< 92 >

Boron and arthritis

Boron may be an effective treatment for arthritis. In areas of the world where boron consumption is 1 mg or less per day, rates of arthritis range from 20 to 70 percent whereas in areas where boron consumption ranges from 3 to 10 mg per day the estimated incidence of arthritis is 0 to 10 percent. A 6 mg boron supplement has been shown to produce a favorable response among 50 percent of subjects with osteoarthritis compared to only 10 percent receiving placebo. [Env Health Pers 102: 83-85, 1994] Daily intake of boron up to 13 mg appears to be safe. [Biol Trace Elem Res 66: 319-30, 1998]

Dietary consumption of boron

Despite its pervasive effect on human health, boron has yet to be declared an essential nutrient. Consumption of 3.25 mg of boron daily even appears to improve brain function. [Env Health Pers 102: 65-72, 1994] Dietary boron consumption ranges from 1 to 4 milligrams per day but a significant portion of the population has very low intake levels, below 1 mg per day. [J Am Dietetic Assn 99: 335, 1999] Raisins and nuts are good dietary sources of boron. It is possible to achieve an intake of 10-30 mg of boron per day from nuts and dried fruits. Thus, boron supplements less than 10 mg would not be considered to be problematic. The safe upper limit for boron is 20 mg per day.

Bottom line: See that your daily multivitamin includes boron, preferably in doses of 3 mg or more per day. Well-made multivitamins will include significant sources of sulfur (taurine, N-acetyl cysteine, alpha lipoic acid, glutathione), coenzyme Q10 and chromium.

< 93 >

Vitamin Truth #9
Balanced Multivitamins

Many nutrients, particularly minerals, must be balanced because they often compete for absorption in the digestive tract and imbalances may result in troublesome health problems. The important minerals to balance in multivitamins are zinc and copper, calcium and magnesium. Carotenoids such as beta carotene and lutein/zeaxanthin must also be balanced. Recent studies also emphasize the need to balance the different forms of vitamin E, the tocopherols and tocotrienols.

Balance the tocopherols and tocotrienols

Family of Vitamin E Molecules	
Tocopherols	**Tocotrienols**
Alpha tocopherol	Alpha tocotrienol
Beta tocopherol	Beta tocotrienol
Delta tocopherol	Delta tocotrienol
Gamma tocopherol	Gamma tocotrienol

Vitamin E is one of the most popular food supplements consumed by Americans. Some vitamin supplement users have been taking vitamin E for decades. Except for two Canadian cardiologists (the Shute brothers) who extolled vitamin E in the 1970s, there weren't many published studies on the health benefits of vitamin E supplements. But the Shute brothers' experience was with adults who have cardiovascular disease, not healthy individuals. Then in 1992-93 it was widely reported that the consumption of 100 IU of vitamin E from diet and supplements reduced the relative risk of coronary heart disease in males and females by 26 and 46 percent respectively over a 2-year period. No benefit was observed from lower doses. [N Eng J Med 328: 1450-56, 1993] A person would have to consume a jar of wheat germ every day to obtain that much vitamin E. Hurray, the long-time vitamin E users were finally

< 94 >

vindicated. Many vitamin E believers were taking 1200 units or more of supplemental vitamin E per day.

Later it was recognized that a significant percentage of Americans simply don't get enough vitamin E. The best diet provides only about 12-15 IU of vitamin E. The Third National Health and Nutrition Examination Survey published in 1999 found <u>30 percent of the US population exhibit low concentrations of vitamin E in blood serum</u>, which would put them at increased risk for heart disease, cancer and other maladies. [Am J Epidem 150: 299-300, 1999] By 1995 it was shown that 100 IU of vitamin E from supplements

> **The body requires tocopherols and tocotrienols**

reduce progression of coronary artery disease in middle-aged males as evidenced by arterial imaging. [J Am Med Assn 273: 1849-54, 1995] In 1996 it was found that vitamin E supplements reduce over-all mortality rates. [Am J Clin Nut 64: 190-96, 1996] In 1997 researchers reported that it takes about 400 IU of vitamin E to keep LDL cholesterol from oxidizing (hardening). [Arterioscler Thromb Vasc Biol 17: 2273-79, 1997] The sales of vitamin E pills boomed to the point where there was a temporary shortage of vitamin E to meet public demand.

Vitamin E protects cholesterol, it doesn't lower cholesterol

In the middle of the craze for vitamin E, critics claimed vitamin E didn't significantly reduce cholesterol. It was bogus criticism since vitamin E rides on cholesterol particles for transport and delivery to various tissues in the body. Reduce cholesterol and there would be less vitamin E supplied to fatty-organs like the brain, eyes, prostate and breast that need extra vitamin E. As cholesterol levels drop in the blood circulation so do levels of vitamin E (tocopherols). As cholesterol drops below 160 mg per deciliter the risk of cancer more than doubles. [Eur Heart J 18: 52-59, 1997] <u>While vitamin E doesn't reduce circulating cholesterol levels, it does keep cholesterol from hardening within blood vessel walls.</u> [Circulation 106: 1453, 2002]

< 95 >

Of recent note, cholesterol is not as strong a predictor of a first-time heart attack or stroke as is elevated levels of C-reactive protein, a marker of inflammation. In one study 77 percent of women who experienced a heart attack or stroke had a total cholesterol count under 160 mg per deciliter of blood which is considered very low. [New Eng J Med 347: 1557-65, 2002] Also of note, both vitamin E and vitamin B6 reduce C-reactive protein levels. [Free Radical Biology Med 29: 790-92, 2000; Circulation 103: 2788, 2001]

Negative studies with high-dose vitamin E

But then things changed. Subsequent studies using vitamin E supplements have been more perplexing. A study of 76,890 nurses for 14 years found that only high intake of vitamin E from foods, not supplements, reduced the risk of Parkinson's disease. [Neurology 59: 1161-69, 2002] Up to 2000 IU of vitamin E taken over an 8-week period by healthy adults produced no reduced markers of cholesterol hardening (lipid peroxidation). [J Am Med Assn 285: 1178-82, 2001] A 300 mg dose of vitamin E taken for 3.5 years did not reduce the risk of stroke or heart attack among adults who has survived a previous heart attack. [Lancet 354: 447-50, 1999] A 300 mg dose of vitamin E among adults with a variety of health problems taken for 3.6 years did not result in a drop in adverse cardiovascular events. [Lancet 357: 89-95, 2001] A 400 IU daily dose of natural-source vitamin E taken by senior adults for a period of 4.5 years also resulted in no reduced risk of stroke or heart attack. [New Eng J Med 342: 154-60, 2000] When these studies are examined together they show some benefit, no effect or slight increased risk for cardiovascular disease among adults. [Nutr Clin Care 5: 50-55, 2002]

Higher doses of vitamin E did not produce health benefits

Another vitamin E study is instructive. In a study of 47,344 males, an intake of 300-500 IU per day of supplemental vitamin E significantly reduced the risk for colon cancer but greater than 600 IU per day

< 96 >

produced no further benefits. [Cancer Epidemiology Biomarkers 11: 1298-304, 2002]

Heart disease prevention requires more than vitamin E

What is the public to make of these negative reports? Have long-time vitamin E users been misdirected? First, while the primary reason why consumers take vitamin E is for the historically-believed cardiovascular benefits, actually there are many more important nutritional factors involved in heart and blood vessel disease than vitamin E, namely folic acid and vitamin B12 in reducing homocysteine levels and magnesium and omega-3 fatty acids from fish or flaxseed oil in reducing the risk of sudden-death heart attack. [Circulation 99: 2452-57, 1999; Circulation 104: 744, 2001; Acta Cardiol 36: 411-29, 1981; Magnesium Trace Elem 9: 143-51, 1990] Approximately 340,000 of the 750,000 annual heart attacks in the US have nothing to do with cholesterol, they involve shortages of magnesium, a natural muscle relaxant, and omega-3 oils. Supplemental vitamin E is beneficial, but not for some of the reasons studied.

Other benefits of vitamin E supplements overlooked

While physicians began to dismiss vitamin E supplements based upon the studies cited above, there were other health benefits that were being overlooked. For example, just 50 mg of vitamin E significantly reduces the relative risk of prostate cancer. [New Eng J Med 330: 1029-35, 1994] Just 200 IU taken by senior adults increases the activity of immune cells by 65 percent. [J Am Med Assoc 277: 1380-86, 1977] Just 50 mg of the alpha tocopherol form of vitamin E has been found to reduce growth factor levels that can hasten the growth of tumors. [Anticancer Research 22: 375-78, 2002] A 200 mg dose of daily vitamin E improved immune response among healthy older adults receiving vaccines for tetanus, pneumococcus, diphtheria and hepatitis B (800 mg/day did not improve immunity better than 200 mg). [J Am Med Assn 277: 1380-86, 1997] The use of 200 IU of daily vitamin E from food supplements has been

< 97 >

shown to produce a *"remarkable decrease systolic blood pressure"* (-24 percent) and diastolic blood pressure (-12.5 percent) as well as reduce the heart rate significantly (-4.3 percent). [Int J Vitamin Nutrition Research, Vol. 10, 2002] Why the quick dismissal of supplemental vitamin E?

Why did most of the studies involving supplemental vitamin E prove to be effective in lower doses, 50-200 IU and not in higher doses, 300-1000 IU? Vitamin E in higher doses than provided from the diet is associated with higher risk of aggressive or fatal prostate cancer in non-smokers. However, this is not true among smokers and individuals with very low intake of vitamin E. [Urology 59: 9-19, 2002] Another large study of 47,780 males also shows high-dose vitamin E (more than 100 IU alpha tocopherol) significantly reduces prostate cancer risk only among smokers and ex-smokers. [Cancer Epidemiology Biomarkers Prev 8: 893-99, 1999] Obviously, smokers have higher need for vitamin E.

Incomplete vitamin E supplements

The answer to this dilemma may be that only one form of vitamin E is provided in most food supplements, the alpha tocopherol form. While studies indicate dietary sources of vitamin E moderately reduce the risk of breast cancer, vitamin E supplements do not. The failing of vitamin E is now believed to be related to the provision of the full family of vitamin E molecules (alpha, beta, delta and gamma tocopherols and tocotrienols). [J Nutr Biochem 13: 2-20, 2002]

The entire vitamin E family consists of four forms of tocopherols and tocotrienols (alpha, beta, delta, gamma). Soybeans, the primary source of natural vitamin E in food supplements, are produced in a manner to isolate the alpha tocopherol form of vitamin E. This is done for good reason. Only alpha tocopherol is found in significant concentration in body tissues 24 hours after ingestion, not the other forms of tocopherols. [Medical Hypotheses 32: 107-10, 1990] Only d-alpha tocopherol exhibits prolonged retention in tissues compared to other forms of vitamin E. However, this may mean the body needs daily supply of the other forms of tocopherols and tocotrienols.

< 98 >

Non-alpha tocopherols

There is a growing body of evidence that non-alpha tocopherols and the tocotrienols may yield health benefits even in small doses and even when not retained in the body for long. Even though gamma tocopherol is only rated to have 10 percent of the biological activity of alpha tocopherol, its presence in the diet is not insignificant. [Am J Clin Nut 27: 980-86, 1974] Gamma tocopherol raises levels of both alpha and gamma tocopherol in blood plasma and it has unique anti-inflammatory properties. In a study of over 10,000 men, those with the highest consumption of gamma tocopherol experienced a significant reduced risk for subsequent prostate cancer and the protective association of selenium and alpha tocopherol were only observed when gamma tocopherol concentrations were high. [J Natl Cancer Institute 92: 2018-23, 2000] While alpha tocopherol inhibits fats from turning rancid in the body, gamma tocopherol is active against nitrogen-induced free radicals that are associated with chronic inflammation.

More about gamma tocopherol

Gamma tocopherol has been found to be superior to alpha tocopherol in inhibiting prostate cancer in laboratory studies. [Seminars Urology Oncology 17: 85-90, 1999] Males who consume the highest amounts of gamma tocopherol from dietary sources appear to have a five-fold reduction in their risk of developing prostate cancer compared to men who consume the lowest amounts. [J Nat Cancer Inst 92: 1966-67, 2000] Recent reviews suggest more attention be given to gamma tocopherol. [Am J Clin Nut 74: 714-22, 2001] Another study shows there was no protection against nonfatal heart attacks among adults who consume the highest dietary amounts of gamma tocopherol. [Epidemiology 13: 216-23, 2002] This does not rule out supplemental gamma tocopherol as being beneficial since even the highest dietary consumption may still be relatively low. In a laboratory study, mixed tocopherols (alpha, beta, delta, gamma) were recently found to be superior to alpha tocopherol

< 99 >

alone in protecting red blood cells from oxidation. [J Cardiovas Pharm 39: 714-21, 2002]

Gamma tocopherol is the predominant tocopherol in the American diet while alpha tocopherol is the form of vitamin E usually provided in multivitamins. Gamma tocopherol appears to be more effective at inhibiting the growth of tumor cells than alpha tocopherol. [FASEB J, Oct 4, 2002]

Enter the tocotrienols

Let's examine the other family of vitamin E molecules, the tocotrienols. Tocotrienols from rice bran have been found to reduce cholesterol when combined with a cholesterol-lowering (statin) drug better than the drug alone. [Atherosclerosis 156: 39-47, 2001] Tocotrienols convert to tocopherols at high doses, so more is not more effective. About 100 mg of tocotrienols is considered the optimal dose. [Atherosclerosis 161: 199-207, 2002] In mice bred for a genetic predisposition toward high cholesterol even when consuming a low-fat diet, the provision of alpha tocopherol reduced atherosclerotic plaques in blood vessels by 11 percent while tocotrienols reduced plaque accumulation by 42 to 47 percent. [J Nutrition 131: 2606-18, 2001]

A recent animal study is telling. Supplementation of rodent diets with alpha tocopherol vitamin E did not improve bone calcium content but provision of vitamin E which included tocopherols and tocotrienols did improve bone calcium content. [Asia Pacific J Clin Nutr 11: 194-99, 2002]

Alpha tocopherol became the vitamin E of choice because it is the only form of this vitamin that is stored in fatty tissues and maintained in the body. [J Nutrition 131: 369S, 2001] However, it is apparent that the daily provision of the other forms of vitamin E, the alpha, beta, delta, gamma tocopherols, even though they are not readily stored in tissues, play an important role in human health. While tocotrienols are inferior compared to alpha tocopherol in regard to retention in tissues, they are

< 100 >

superior antioxidants. Make sure your vitamin pill provides 75 to 100 percent of the alpha form of vitamin E along with an array of the other tocopherols and tocotrienols. It's more important that your vitamin E is produced from a natural source, like soy, and that it is provided in the highly absorbable dry powered form (succinate). [Arteriosclerosis, Thrombosis, Vascular Biology 17: 2273-79, 1997]

Furthermore, vitamin E works in tandem with the trace mineral selenium to produce an important antioxidant enzyme (glutathione peroxidase) that protects fats in the body from spoiling. [Nutritional Biochemistry 9: 23-27, 1998]

Bottom line: Scientific studies are expanding our knowledge of vitamin E molecules to include <u>the family of tocopherols and tocotrienols which produce health benefits</u>. The higher the dose of alpha tocopherol the less effective it was in some studies. Recognizing a change in the scientific understanding of how vitamin E works, the *Berkeley Wellness Letter* has lowered their recommendation for supplemental vitamin E to 200-400 IU per day (instead of up to 800 IU). [Berkeley Wellness Letter, Sept. 1999] It's probably more important to include the full family of mixed (alpha, beta, delta, gamma) tocopherols and tocotrienols as well as provide the predominant form of vitamin E stored in the body, alpha tocopherol. Furthermore, vitamin E is not complete without accompanying selenium which may be low in soils in some geographical areas of the US. <u>Probably 200-300 IU of d-alpha tocopherol is an optimal dose accompanied by mixed tocopherols and tocotrienols.</u>

Zinc and Copper must be balanced

Zinc and copper are in delicate balance with each other in the human body. Both of these minerals are essential for human health. These minerals compete for absorption and when zinc consumption exceeds copper by a factor of ten, then there may be a buildup of LDL "bad" cholesterol in the blood circulation. [The Right Dose, P. Hausman, Ballantine Books, 1991] Some vitamin pills designed for eye conditions provide 40 mg of zinc in each pill accompanied by a small amount of

< 101 >

copper. Some adults with retinal disease take two pills per day and thus get 80 mg of zinc and only 2-4 mg of copper. Many of these people exhibit high cholesterol levels and never realize their vitamin pill may be the cause of the problem. Researchers at the University of Kentucky suggest zinc consumption not exceed 25 mg per day. [Zinc metabolism in the elderly, Geriatric Nutrition, Raven Press, 1990]

Even though it is an essential mineral, most Americans consume small amounts of copper, about 1.3 mg, from tap water or plant foods. [Advance Data, Natl Center for Health Statistics No. 258, Nov. 14, 1994] Excessive amounts of copper may induce health problems. **Bottom line:** The best way to maintain a healthy zinc/copper ratio is to consume no more than 15-25 mg of zinc from a daily multivitamin and obtain copper from the diet.

Balancing the Major Minerals		
Minerals/ daily dietary intake	**Re-balance point**	**Imbalance leads to**
Sodium ~4000 mg per day; Potassium ~3000 mg/day	Americans need 500-1000 mg added potassium to daily diet; sodium should be limited	Hypertension, bone loss
Calcium ~800 mg per day; Magnesium 200-275 mg per day	Americans may need 400 mg magnesium added to daily diet for proper cal-mag balance	Sudden-death heart attack; muscle spasm, leg cramps, anxiety reactions
Zinc ~10 mg; copper 1-2 mg	Zinc supplement greater than 25 mg need to be accompanied by 2 mg copper; ratio should be 10-to-1 zinc over copper	Excessive zinc without copper leads to rise in cholesterol

< 102 >

The Calcium/Magnesium Ratio
Caution: Imbalance is harmful

Calcium is the most widely promoted mineral supplement, endorsed by health authorities far and wide. Health authorities who have traditionally been reluctant to recommend food supplements have had no qualms about supplemental calcium. American women are now being advised by the National Institutes of Health to consume 1200-1500 mg of calcium daily to avoid thinning of the bones (osteoporosis) in the later years of life. Women have increased their consumption of calcium by 56 percent in the past decade. [J Can Dietetic Association 58: 77-83, 1997]

Some women, believing more calcium is better, consume 3000+ mg of daily calcium from the diet plus supplements. Researchers indicate adverse effects of high-calcium diets may occur at intakes greater than 2000 mg per day. High-dose calcium interferes with the absorption of other minerals such as zinc and magnesium. [Nutrition Reviews 55: 1-9, 1997] In countries where milk consumption is high, the incidence of high blood pressure increases with advancing age. Milk is a rich source of calcium. [Int'l Journal Cardiology 33: 191-98, 1991] The mortality rates of males under 50 years of age doubles with increased levels of calcium in the blood stream. [J Clinical Endocrinology & Metabolism 81: 2149-53, 1996]

> *Most Americans are mistakenly advised to consume more and more calcium*

Americans consume far too much calcium from the diet, in a four-to-one ratio over magnesium. Side effects from too much calcium begin when a person consumes calcium in a ratio of five-to-one over magnesium. Finland has the highest ratio of calcium intake over magnesium, 7-to-1, and has the highest rate of heart and blood vessel disease in the world. [J Am College Nutrition 13: 429-46, 1994]

< 103 >

Due to hormonal changes, women are losing calcium from their bones, particularly after age 40. Pressure was applied to health authorities to do something about the rising rate of hip fractures and mortality rates among older females. The quick answer was to increase the Recommended Daily Allowance for calcium from 800 to 1500 mg per day since calcium is the major mineral in bone. This may have been a big mistake.

The National Institutes of Health indicates many Americans fall short of achieving optimal calcium intake. Here is the advice given to women. Women between the ages of 25-50 years should get 1000 mg of calcium per day and after age 65, 1500 mg per day. Males should get about 1000 mg per day. An upper limit of 2000 mg per day appears to be safe for most individuals, say researchers. [NIH Consensus Statement 12: 1-31, 1994] The National Academy of Sciences says the overdose point is 2500 mg per day. The problem here is that the *"safe"* upper limit of 2000-2500 milligrams can be troublesome.

Do we need to take calcium supplements?

Bone/mineral formulas often provide 100 percent of the daily need for calcium, 1200-1500 mg, in their products with no consideration for dietary intake. Dietary calcium consumption for middle-aged women is about 750 mg and for older women about 650 mg. Millions of women consume more than 2000 mg of calcium from diet and supplements and are over-dosing on calcium. Adverse effects from calcium (diet plus supplements) begin at 2000 mg per day. [Nutrition Reviews 55: 1, 1997; Am J Clin Nut 65: 1803, 1997] What are the consequences?

Calcium affects more than bones

Calcium is not just for bones. Calcium and magnesium help to produce muscle tone. Calcium constricts and magnesium relaxes smooth muscles. An oversupply of calcium accompanied by a shortage of magnesium would result in muscle spasm, which is frequently experienced by people

< 104 >

who over-dose on calcium. Common symptoms are migraines, eyelid twitch, heart flutters, backache, leg cramps, anxiety, toe cramping, constipation and monthly cramping in females. An example of the muscle balancing between calcium and magnesium is regularity. Too much calcium and the bowels will be tight (constipation). Too much magnesium and you will be too regular (loose stool). [Haematologica 83: 118, 1998; Acta Paediatrica Scand 80: 964, 1991]

> ## Calcium lost from bones accumulates elsewhere

Combine the fixation on calcium consumption with the fact the American diet provides far too little magnesium, and you've got a major public health problem. Most troublesome, the widespread shortage of magnesium is directly related to sudden heart spasm, the heart being a large muscle pump. An estimated 340,000 of the 750,000 heart attacks that occur annually in the US are attributed to a lack of magnesium. The more that calcium dominates over magnesium the greater the risk for sudden death heart attack. [Science 208: 198, 1980]

Where's the lost calcium going?

That's not all. As calcium is being lost from bones due to hormonal changes it is being deposited in arteries and other organs. How does flooding the body with more calcium stop this? Women with osteoporosis have a high risk of developing blood vessel disease. [Calcified Tissue Intl 62: 209-13, 1998] A CAT scan is commonly performed to detect calcium deposits in arteries. Calcium can also accumulate in the kidneys as stones (1 in 11 Americans) and in the heart (mitral) valve (1 in 12 Americans). Do you still want to keep taking all that calcium? The highest mortality rates in the world occur in countries that consume the most calcium from dairy products (New Zealand, North America, Scandinavian countries). [Int J Cardiol 33: 19, 1991] Even when dairy fat is removed (non-fat milk) there is a strong association between calcium and coronary heart disease among men over age 45 and females over age 75. [Alt Med Review 3: 281: 1998] Among men less than 50 years of age, high blood calcium

< 105 >

levels are associated with a 30 to 200 percent increase in mortality from cardiovascular disease. [J Clin Endocrin Metab 81: 2149, 1996]

All-cause Mortality Rate and Daily Consumption of Calcium-rich Milk Protein		
Country	Mortality rate per 100,000 population ages 55-64 years	Consumption of calcium-rich milk protein (excluding cheese)
Finland	686	37.8 grams
Ireland	692	29.3 grams
Denmark	568	22.8 grams
Norway	560	25.1 grams
United States	421	15.8 grams
Germany	366	13.9 grams
Italy	268	8.7 grams
Portugal	208	6.3 grams
Japan	63	4.4 grams
Ref: Intl J Cardiology 33:19, 1991		

Calcium and cancer

Calcium does not increase cancer incidence and dietary or supplemental calcium may help prevent colon cancer. [Nutrition Cancer 41: 150-55, 2001] The consumption of a moderate amount of calcium (700-800 mg from foods or supplements, about what is consumed from the typical American diet) decreases the relative risk of colon cancer compared to calcium intake below 500 mg per day. [J Natl Cancer Inst 94: 437-46, 2002] But elevated calcium levels increase the risk of dying from cancer by 58 percent. [J Clin Endocrin Metab 81: 2149, 1996] Women who maintain strong bones appear to be at greater risk to develop breast cancer. Postmenopausal women on hormone replacement therapy who have high bone mineral density scores experience a significant increase in risk for breast cancer. [Environmental Health Perspectives 105: 593, 1997] Micro-calcifications develop in malignant breast disease. [British J Radiology 70: 375, 1997]

< 106 >

Calcium and arteries

Either high dietary calcium intake with no supplemental calcium, or supplemental calcium with low-dietary intake, appears to reduce the risk of cardiovascular problems. [Am J Epidemiology 149: 151, 1999] Americans are being advised to do both, acquire more calcium from foods and supplements.

When animals are given diets where sodium predominates over potassium, and calcium over magnesium, ninety percent of the animals die within 5-7 weeks. When these mineral imbalances are corrected, only 19 percent die in the same time period. [Electrolytes Cardiovas Disease, S. Karger, 1965] In the American diet, sodium and calcium predominate.

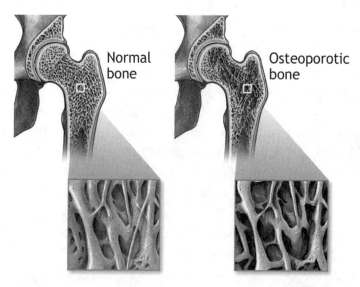

Normal bone

Osteoporotic bone

⚘A.D.A.M.

Bone density is not the only marker of bone integrity. Pure calcium crystals produce brittle bones. Magnesium interferes with crystallization and produces flexible bones that can withstand physical stress. Boron, a trace mineral, enhances bone hardness.

< 107 >

Calcium doesn't arrest bone loss

It's true, starting at about age 40 for females, and about age 50 for males, there is about a 1 percent loss of bone density per year thereafter. This can eventually result in fractures of the bones in the neck, back, wrist and hip. But most of the studies show that calcium supplements don't reverse bone loss they only slow down the rate of bone loss. A 1993 study showed that 760-1000 milligrams of supplemental calcium daily reduces the rate of bone loss significantly, but still the rate was only slowed, not stopped. [New Eng J Med 328: 460, 1993] Another report admits calcium supplementation slows the rate of bone loss by 30 to 50 percent but *"does not completely arrest postmenopausal bone loss."* [Am J Med 312: 278-86, 1996] Postmenopausal females who take calcium supplements should not be surprised when their bone density test reveals declining bone mass. Calcium alone does not add bone mass.

Sodium inhibits calcium absorption

Calcium deficiency cannot be the sole reason why American women exhibit a high rate of bone loss (osteoporosis). Women in Asian countries only consume about 400 mg of calcium per day and have far fewer hip fractures and a much lower mortality rate. Hip fractures are only about 247 per 100,000 women in Hong Kong and 535 per 100,000 women in the USA. [Am J Clin Nut 70: 539S, 1999] American women consume up to 4000 mg of sodium per day versus 1500 mg per day in Japan. Sodium competes with calcium for absorption and impairs the availability of calcium. This is why Americans need more calcium to keep their bones strong than do Asians.

Beyond calcium

Furthermore, Americans are solely fixated on calcium to increase bone density. Nutrients such as magnesium, boron, vitamin C, vitamin D, vitamin K, vitamin B6 and folic acid combined with salt and protein

< 108 >

restriction and physical exercise should be emphasized. [British J Biomed Sci 51: 228-40, 1994; J Am College Nut 19: 715-37, 2000]

Does magnesium increase bone mass?

<u>Women are never told that magnesium also strengthens bones</u>. [Medical Tribune, July 22, 1993; Mineral Electrolyte Metabolism 24: 314-20, 1998] A diet low in magnesium results in loss of bone mineral density. [J Bone Min Res 10: 466, 1995] In 1988 Dutch researchers theorized that a magnesium deficiency was the real cause of osteoporosis and calcifications throughout the body. [Ned Tijdschr Tandheelkd 100: 413-14, 1993] In a small study

Magnesium alone increases bone density

of 19 women, 15 who had low bone mineral density that made them prone to fractures, within one year on magnesium supplements only 7 of the 19 women still had low bone mineral levels. [J Reproductive Med 35: 503, 1990] While magnesium interferes somewhat with the absorption of calcium, it promotes bone formation and prevents loss of bone and increases bone strength. [J Nutrition 130: 216-20, 2000] The provision of 245 to 800 mg of magnesium per day has not been found to adversely affect calcium balance. [Clinics Geriatric Med 3: 389, 1987] <u>Israeli researchers solely prescribed 250-750 mg of magnesium to postmenopausal females and 71 percent experienced a 1 to 8 percent rise in bone density</u>. [Magnesium Res 6: 155, 1993] Calcium crystals will produce brittle bones. Magnesium interrupts the crystallization of calcium and produces flexible, elastic bones. [J Am College Nut 12: 442, 1993; Cal Tissue Res 23: 245-50, 1977]

The provision of 250-300 mg of supplemental magnesium over a 2-year period increased bone density among 71 percent of postmenopausal women with chronic back pain due to osteoporosis. [Nutrition Reviews 53: 71-80, 1995]

The American Dairy Council recommends calcium-rich dairy products for bone health but these foods provide very little magnesium. While

< 109 >

dairy products are high in calcium, about 25 percent of the American adult population is lactose intolerant and cannot easily digest dairy products. [New Eng J Med 333: 1, 1995] It can take a year to restore adequate magnesium levels. [Pediatric Asthma, Allergy & Immun 5: 273, 1991]

This information is going to be perplexing to Americans who take calcium supplements, after all, as they often are taking these supplements under the watchful eye of their personal physician and the recommendation of the National Institutes of Health.

| Progressive Decline in Dietary Magnesium ||
Years	Magnesium intake, milligrams per day
1900-1908	475-500 mg
1909-1913	415-435 mg
1925-1929	385-398 mg
1935-1939	360-375 mg
1947-1949	358-370 mg
1957-1959	340-360 mg
1965-1976	300-340 mg
1978-1985	225-318 mg
1990	175-225 mg
1988-1994	231-376 mg
Sources: Magnesium Trace Elements 10: 182, 92, 1991; Vital & Health Statistics, Series 11, No. 245, 2002	

Magnesium for health

Magnesium supplements have wide ranging health benefits. Supplemental magnesium appears to reduce calcium deposits, as evidenced by reduced calcium stone formation in the kidneys. [J Urology 159: 669, 1998; 124: 779, 1980] Supplemental magnesium has been shown to eliminate irregular heart beats after heart bypass surgery. [Nippon Kyobu Ceka Gakkai Zasshi 46: 287, 1996] Magnesium, 600 mg per day, decreases the frequency of migraine headaches. [Cephalgia 16: 257, 1996]

< 110 >

Calcium, magnesium ratio

Calcium must be balanced with magnesium. Low magnesium levels, and high calcium levels, predispose men to sudden death heart attack and stroke as well as calcifications throughout the body. [Science 208: 198-200, 1980; Magnesium 1: 277-91, 1982; Calcified Tissue Internatl 32: 139-43, 1980] A compelling study conducted by the US Department of Agriculture found that abnormal heart beats are more common as magnesium intake is reduced in the diet and that most women who eat less food than males do not consume the recommended 280 mg (US RDA 1989) of magnesium. The use of caffeine, water pills (diuretics), estrogen and infection increase the need for magnesium and put many people in the population at risk for heart rhythm abnormalities. [Am J Clin Nut 75: 550-54, 2002]

The 2-to-1 ratio of calcium over magnesium, provided in most mineral formulas, may need to be adjusted. It was crudely developed decades ago based upon the fact the body has twice as much calcium and magnesium by weight. This ratio of calcium to magnesium may not be ideal for optimal health. The concurrent use of calcium and estrogen supplements in postmenopausal females may lead to heightened states of anxiety and blood clotting. [Magnesium Research 3: 197-215, 1990]

The American diet provides calcium in about a 2.5 to 1.0 ratio over magnesium. Calcium supplements to prevent osteoporosis could throw the calcium to magnesium ratio above the 4-to-1 figure in Finland, the country with the highest heart disease death rate for young to middle-aged men. [J Am College Nut 13: 429, 1994] Probably Americans should consume more equal ratios of calcium and magnesium.

Does magnesium interfere with the absorption of calcium?

There is a false idea that magnesium interferes with the absorption of calcium. Increasing magnesium intake up to 826 milligrams per day

< 111 >

was not found to inhibit calcium absorption at an intake level of 812 milligrams of calcium. [Journal American College Nutrition, Volume 13, 1994]

	Recommended Daily Intake Diet + Supplements	Typical daily dietary intake	Typical amount in bone/mineral supplements
Calcium (muscle tightener)	1200	866-1208 mg	1000-1200 mg
Magnesium (muscle relaxant)	400	231-376 mg	400-500 mg
Ratio of calcium over magnesium	4 to 1	3 to 1	2 to 1

	Total daily consumption food + supplements	Overdose point where adverse symptoms may occur
Calcium (muscle tightener)	1866-2408 mg	2000 mg (muscle spasm)
Magnesium (muscle relaxant)	631-876 mg	Depends upon ratio to calcium (loose stool)
Ratio of calcium over magnesium	3 to 1	4 to 1

Calcium absorption

The provision of more and more calcium to avoid bone loss with advancing age has its drawbacks. About 75 percent of older women have significant problems absorbing calcium from foods or supplements. Since vitamin D regulates calcium absorption, it is no surprise that 60 percent of women with bone thinning have low vitamin D levels. Vitamin D thwarts bone loss in two ways: (1) by preventing overproduction of parathyroid hormones that accelerate bone loss with advancing age;

< 112 >

(2) increasing absorption of calcium from foods and supplements. By maintaining adequate vitamin D levels, the need for calcium is cut in half. When adequate levels of vitamin D are maintained, the need for calcium is reduced to 800 mg per day. The incidence of calcium overload from vitamin D supplements (1000 IU per day) is very low and is usually caused by excessive calcium intake. [J Rheumatology 23: 15, 1996]

Form of calcium	Tablet strength	Number of tablets for 1000 mg of elemental calcium	Amount elemental calcium by percent	Amount elemental calcium by weight per tablet
Calcium carbonate (relatively insoluble)	625 mg	4	40%	250 mg
Calcium citrate (More soluble; requires no stomach acid for absorption)	950 mg	5	21%	200 mg
Calcium gluconate	500 mg	22	9%	45 mg
Calcium lactate	325 mg	24	13%	42 mg

When to take calcium supplements

The National Institutes of Health suggests that adults consume calcium supplements in divided doses, between meals, up to 500 mg, since there are mechanisms in the human body that inhibit calcium absorption beyond this amount. However, calcium absorption is optimal when the stomach is acidic, that is, when food is being consumed. Low stomach acid levels between meals do not facilitate absorption of calcium carbonate.

Up to 30 percent of older adults do not produce sufficient amounts of gastric acid, and thus their absorption of calcium may be impaired.). [Public Health Reports, 104: 46-50 1989] Individuals with low stomach

< 113 >

acid may absorb less than 2 percent of their dietary calcium. In one study, individuals with normal stomach acid absorbed about 24 percent of calcium citrate and carbonate, but when the supply of stomach acid was low only 5 percent of calcium carbonate was absorbed compared to 40 to 45 percent of calcium citrate. [Nutrition Reviews 52: 221, 1994]

It's best to take calcium citrate supplements, which do not require stomach acid for absorption, in between meals.

Common Forms of Calcium in Food Supplements	
Calcium carbonate	Most common form of calcium provided in food supplements. Needs to be taken with a meal to be absorbed properly. May not be absorbed well by older adults who do not produce sufficient amounts of stomach acid or take acid blockers to control heartburn. Health authorities recommend taking calcium supplements in between meals when stomach acid levels are low.
Calcium citrate	Does not require stomach acid for absorption. Exhibits superior absorption.

Form of calcium

Most popular brands of multivitamins provide calcium carbonate which neutralizes gastric acid and most of it is excreted undissolved. Calcium citrate is absorbed regardless of the availability of digestive juice and minimizess the formation of kidney stones. [Food Technology, June 1996] Calcium from oyster shell, dolomite or bone meal may contain toxic metals (lead). Calcium citrate is preferred. Likewise, studies show that magnesium oxide is poorly absorbed (4 percent absorption) and other forms of magnesium would be more desirable (citrate, chloride, lactate, aspartate, etc.) [Magnesium Research 14: 257-62, 2001]

< 114 >

Calcium citrate appears to be superior to calcium carbonate, particularly when following the advice to take calcium supplements between meals. [J Bone Mineral Res 3: 253, 1988] Furthermore, calcium citrate does not appear to induce kidney stone formation. [J Endocrinology Metabolism 61: 1223, 1985] Even though calcium citrate is a highly absorbed form of this mineral, a recent study showed that the bioavailability of calcium citrate and carbonate were similar among women being given estrogen-replacement supplements. Estrogen status and vitamin D appear to be more important than the form of calcium supplement in regards to absorption. [J Clinical Pharmacology 42: 1251-56, 2002] In this regard, refer to the section in this book on boron and its role in helping to maintain hormone levels.

Nutrients to look for in a bone mineral formula	To be used in addition to a well-designed multivitamin The following nutrients have been shown to improve bone density, flexibility and hardness. Dosage range
Vitamin C	200 mg +
Vitamin D3	1000-4000 IU (textbooks are in error on overdose point for vitamin D)
Vitamin K	100-150 mcg (check with doctor if using blood thinners)
Calcium	400-600 mg (assumes 800 mg of calcium is obtained from the diet) Look for citrate form which requires no stomach acid for absorption
Magnesium	400-600 mg
Boron	3-8 mg

Bottom line: The bulkiness of calcium and magnesium requires they be taken separately from multivitamins. Adults need no more than 400-600 mg of supplemental calcium per day to add to a typical calcium-rich American diet (~800 mg) to reach the recommended total daily intake of 1200-1500 mg per day. Supplements are superior to calcium-rich dairy products which may, because of lactose intolerance, induce symptoms of indigestion. For optimal utilization, calcium supplements should be

< 115 >

limited to no more than 500 mg doses taken in between meals. Calcium citrate requires no stomach acid for absorption and is the preferred form of calcium, particularly for adults with absorption problems. Calcium should be balanced with near-equal amounts of magnesium to prevent muscle cramping, sudden-heart muscle spasm, calcifications and other undesirable effects. Bone building regimens should not be centered on calcium alone but should include foods and supplements that provide an array of nutrients including calcium, magnesium, boron and vitamins C, D, K.

Mix the colors: the carotenoids

Most Americans have heard of beta carotene, the orange plant pigment that has been widely touted for its ability to fight cancer. Beta carotene is commonly found in tuberous vegetables such as carrots, sweet potatoes, yams, pumpkin, and cantaloupes. Beta carotene is converted to vitamin A in the liver. Beta carotene belongs to a family of plant pigments called carotenoids. While there are hundreds of known carotenoids, the three major carotenoid plant pigments in the diet are beta carotene (orange), lycopene (red) and lutein/zeaxanthin (yellow).

US Department of Agriculture researchers suggest that lutein and lycopene are the predominant carotenoid pigments in plant food diets, with beta carotene a distant third. [Report, US Dept. of Agriculture Food Composition Laboratory, 1997]

While dietary sources of these antioxidant plant pigments are desired, studies show that supplements have unique advantages. For example, beta carotene in supplements is absorbed much better than from foods. [J Nutrition 130: 503-06, 2000] While a carrot provides about 10,000 IU of vitamin A activity from beta carotene, very little beta carotene is absorbed due to its high fiber content. [J Nutrition 129: 2170-76, 1999] Here again, supplements may be superior to foods.

< 116 >

Plant Pigments	Found in	Promote health in target tissues
Beta carotene (orange)	Yams, sweet potatoes, carrots, squash, cantaloupe	Skin, retards oxidation of cholesterol
Lutein/zeaxanthin (yellow)	Kale, spinach, wolfberry	Retina (macula), lungs, skin
Lycopene (red)	Tomatoes, watermelon	Prostate gland

Carotenoid balance

When the consumption of carotenoids is high, and the intake of lutein and zeaxanthin are not exceeded by beta carotene, health benefits are achieved. In the Fiji Islands the incidence of lung cancer among male smokers has almost disappeared because Fiji Islanders use taro root, hibiscus leaf and wild spinach leaves to wrap their food. These are carotenoid-rich plant foods which provide more lutein and zeaxanthin than beta carotene. In other South Pacific Islands where the consumption of beta carotene exceeds that of lutein, the incidence of lung cancer among smokers remains high. [Internat'l J Cancer 63: 18-23, 1995] In one study high-dose (50 mg) beta carotene was ineffective in preventing lung cancer, which could be explained by the lack of lutein. [J Nat'l Cancer Institute 88: 1560-70, 1996]

Carotenoid pigments such as beta carotene, lycopene and lutein/zeaxanthin require a small amount of fat in a meal to be absorbed, however lutein requires a bit more fat to achieve the same absorption. [Am J Clin Nut 71: 1187-93, 2000] These colored pigments compete for absorption, so they need to be balanced in multivitamin formulas. [Am J Clin Nut 75: 526-34, 2002]

Regretably, most daily multivitamins provide beta carotene and little or no lutein. A growing number of multivitamin brands are adding lutein, but only a small amount, not enough to make up for dietary shortages. A widely promoted "natural" carotenoid mixture (Betatene-Henkel)

< 117 >

provides a miniscule amount of lutein and zeaxanthin. Beta carotene competes with lutein for absorption. [Am J Clinical Nutrition 55: 1120-25, 1992]

Health benefits of lutein/zeaxanthin

Researchers are just now beginning to report on the importance of lutein and zeaxanthin in the prevention of breast cancer [Journal Nutrition 128: 1650-56, 1998] and retinal disease. People who do not regularly consume dark-green leafy vegetables such as spinach and kale, which are rich natural sources of lutein and zeaxanthin, have been found to be at greater risk to develop retinal disease (macular degeneration). It takes at least 6 mg of lutein per day to reduce the risk of macular degeneration by 57 percent. [J Am Medical Assn 272: 1413-20, 1994] Dr. Stuart Richer of the Veterans Medical Center in North Chicago, Illinois, has demonstrated that the provision of lutein supplements may reverse some of the visual deficits (blind spots, glare problems) experienced by macular disease patients in just a few months. [J Am Optom Assoc. 70: 24-36, 1999]

Get a full six milligrams of supplemental lutein

It takes about five servings of spinach per week to consume that much lutein. Up to 30 percent of adults show early signs of retinal deterioration by the age of 30 and 9 percent of older Americans have lost some central vision due to retinal degeneration.

One study reveals that 60-year-old individuals who maintain adequate levels of lutein and zeaxanthin in the retinas of their eyes exhibit the visual sensitivity of 20-year olds! [Invest Ophthalmology Visual Science 39: 397-406, 1998] Retinal levels of lutein decline with advancing age and a recent study found macular degeneration patients had 32 percent less lutein than old adults with healthy eyes. A 4 milligram lutein supplement taken after a diagnosis of macular degeneration will restore retinal lutein levels to levels found in healthy eyes. [Ophthalmology 109: 1780-87, 2002] By consuming vitamin pills that only provide beta

< 118 >

carotene and no lutein, health-conscious Americans may unwittingly hasten on the day when their retina becomes weak and they lose some of their central vision. Blue-green and hazel-eyed individuals are 20 times more prone to develop retinal disease because their eyes have half as much lutein and zeaxanthin pigments.

Of interest is the recent finding that individuals who have more body fat may store more lutein in their body tissues and this may impair delivery of lutein and zeaxanthin to the retina. [Investigative Ophthalmology 43: 47-50, 2002] This is particularly true among females who have a higher risk for retinal disease. [Am J Clin Nut 71: 1555-62, 2000]

Researchers have found that lutein/zeaxanthin is far better absorbed (40 percent higher) from spinach and eggs than from food supplements. [Tufts University Health & Nutrition Newsletter, Dec. 2002] But an egg only provides about 300 micrograms of lutein and 1 cup servings of spinach about 3.6 to 12.6 mg of lutein/zeaxanthin. It would still require quite a few servings of these lutein/zeaxanthin-rich foods to equal the weekly amount (about 42 mg) found to reduce the risk of macular degeneration. Furthermore, since beta carotene is provide in virtually all multivitamins, lutein needs to be included in food supplements to provide for carotenoid balance.

Lycopene more economical from foods

The health benefits of lycopene, the red pigment found in watermelon, red grapefruits and tomatoes, are now becoming better known. [Canadian Med Assoc J 163, 2000] Dietary consumption of lycopene averages about 6 milligrams per day and up to 13 milligrams per day in males. High dietary intake of lycopene-rich tomato products has been shown to reduce the risk of

Catsup provides more lycopene than pills

prostate cancer by 30 to 40 percent in 5 studies. In the largest relevant dietary study conducted among male health professionals, just 2 to 4 servings of tomato sauce per week was associated with a 35 percent risk

< 119 >

reduction for prostate cancer (and a 50 percent reduction for advanced prostate cancer). [Exp Biol Med 227: 852-59, 2002] In a supplement study, a 30 mg lycopene pill has been shown to be helpful in shrinking prostate tumors in males. [Exp Biol Med 227: 881-85, 2002] However, the consumption of tomato sauce-based pasta among prostate cancer patients, providing 30 mg of lycopene per day, has been demonstrated to achieve similar results at far less cost. [Exp Biol Med 227: 886-93, 2002] Dietary sources of lycopene are far more cost effective. Simply stated, lycopene is far too costly as an extracted pigment from tomatoes, to be added to multivitamins. Bring on the pasta sauce!

Sources of Lycopene		
Tomato juice	1 cup	20 mg
Tomato puree	1/2 cup	18 mg
Tomato sauce	1/2 cup	17 mg
Tomato soup	1 cup	12 mg
Tomato	Fresh	12 mg
Tomato catsup	2 tblespns	5 mg
Lycopene supplement	1 softgel	5-15 mg (30-day supply $10-16 retail price)

< 120 >

Bottom line: A well-balanced daily multivitamin should provide ample amounts of lutein/zeaxanthin and beta carotene, preferably in equal amounts. Lutein is always accompanied by a small amount of zeaxanthin in nature. Food supplements that provide lutein will always have some accompanying zeaxanthin, though the latter is not always included on labels. Labels which indicate a multivitamin provides both lutein and zeaxanthin aren't necessarily superior to those brands only labelled to provide lutein. In regard to multivitamins, lycopene is best acquired from the diet rather than pills.

< 121 >

Vitamin Truth #10
Do We Need Everything They Put In Multivitamins?

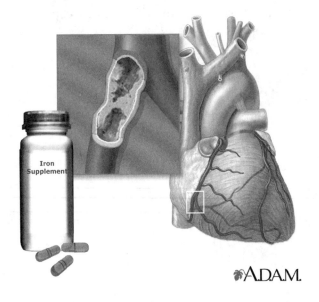

Iron stored in the body over time may increase the risk of disease, particularly heart and liver disease. Iron supplements are not recommended for full grown males, postmenopausal females or women who have undergone early hysterectomy.

Less iron as we grow older

Iron is essential for proper cell growth and for hemoglobin in red blood cells. Trouble is, studies show we may well be ingesting too much iron in the last half of life. Studies show that high iron stores in the body increse the risk of several chronic diseases. Health authorities now say that that *"unprescribed use of supplemental iron by elderly Americans on a Western-style diet is unnecessary."* [Am J Clin Nut 76: 1375, 2002] Recognize

< 122 >

that foods in the US are fortified with iron, which runs contrary to this advice.

This is not to say that supplemental iron may not be needed from time to time. Children certainly need iron to produce more red blood cells as they grow. By the way, an increase in consumption of vitamin C in foods or supplements will increase the absorption of iron from foods. A major cause of mental lethargy among children is the lack of iron due to the lack of oxygen-carrying red blood cells to the brain. Children who under-perform in school should not be placed on stimulant drugs (Ritalin) for attention-deficit disorder, but rather be given a trial course of supplemental vitamin C and/or iron. In one study, 14 boys, ages 7-11 years, who exhibited attention deficits and hyperactivity, showed improvement when given an iron supplement. An iron supplement improved behavior within 30 days. [Neuropsychobiology 35: 178-80, 1997]

Pregnant and menstruating females also have high iron needs. Symptoms such as cold hands and feet, fatigue and pale skin may be signs of overt iron deficiency.

On the other hand, full-grown males begin to accumulate iron at the rate of about 1 milligram per day of life after age 18 or so. A 45-year old male will have twice the iron level as a female of the same age and twice the rate of infection, cancer, diabetes and heart disease. [Eur J Clin Nut 52: 623, 1998] Females outlive males by about eight years

Avoid supplemental iron in full-grown males and post-menopausal females

on average which is attributed to their lower iron stores. Once women cease having a monthly cycle or undergo an early hysterectomy they too begin to accumulate excess iron and do not require iron supplements. Foods are fortified with iron, so certainly no iron pills should be taken by adults in the retirement years. [Iron Time Bomb, B Sardi, 2000]

< 123 >

The only safe form of iron pills that should be consumed and stored at home is carbonyl iron (trade name Ferronyl- BASF). Ferronyl is 98 percent elemental iron. Just 18 mg of Ferronyl (carbonyl) iron is equivalent to 54.4 mg of ferrous fumarate and 150 mgs of ferrous gluconate, other forms of iron commonly used in food supplements. Ferronyl has recently been demonstrated to be two to three times more bioavailable and more effective in elevating red blood cell (hemoglobin) levels than other forms of iron powder (ferrous sulfate). [US Dept. Agriculture] Ferronyl has a long history of safety, having been given to animals in large doses (10,000 mg) without side effects. It is also far less irritating to the digestive tract (no nausea) and does not induce constipation. Ferronyl iron does not cause the potential lethal toxicity associated with inadvertant childhood overdose. The poison control centers report that among young children who overdosed on iron pills, 82 percent who took carbonyl organic iron did not require hospitalization and the remaining children only required observation in an emergency room. Serious toxicity did not occur. [Vet Hum Toxicology 44: 28, 2002] The widespread use of carbonyl iron may prevent the mortal cases of iron overdose that occur among young children annually. Throw out any iron pills, other than Ferronyl, you have at home.

Only Ferronyl (carbonyl) iron is safe

Many vitamin pills provide 10-18 mg of iron. The diet provides an additional 11-13 mg. Iron consumption in the last decade has risen by 56 percent. [Townsend Letter for Doctors, Oct. '98] It is generally believed that many Americans don't get enough iron. Red meats provide ample amounts of iron in a very absorbable form. Growing children and pregnant, lactating and menstruating females may need extra iron. About 80 percent of iron resides in the blood circulation. Due to menstruation, women have half the blood levels of iron compared to men and exhibit half the rate of cancer, diabetes and heart disease. There is no outlet for iron to be purged from the blood circulation in males and by age 50 men may have 20,000-30,000 mg of excess iron in their circulation. [Whole Foods, June '98] After age 40 males accumulate

< 124 >

THE NEW TRUTH ABOUT VITAMINS & MINERALS

one excess milligram of iron per day of life. Ditto for women having undergone early hysterectomy.

<u>Females experience less heart disease and cancer compared to males until women reach menopause when their iron levels begin to rise.</u> We now know that adults who regularly donate blood, and thus have lower iron levels, are healthier. Blood letting to reduce excessive levels of iron and copper is now being considered as a treatment for cancer, heart disease, Parkinson's and Alzheimer's disease and diabetes.

Recent studies show that adults who consume more iron in their diet increase their risk of heart disease. <u>For every one mg of dietary iron, the risk of heart disease increases by about 5 percent.</u> [New England J Med 330: 1152, 1994] Studies like these have caused a number of vitamin companies to remove iron from the adult multivitamin pills. <u>For adults, iron should be acquired solely from the diet.</u> Since the 1st multivitamin survey recommended avoidance of iron in fortified foods and supplements for full-grown males and postmenopausal females, the Institutes of Medicine now suggests adult males and postmenopausal females avoid iron supplements and highly fortified foods. [Nutrition Clinical Care 5: 236-50, 2002] <u>To counter iron buildup in the blood circulation, iron-binding antioxidants should be consumed daily.</u> Bioflavonoids, like cranberry, bilberry, blueberry, quercetin, lemon, grape seed, green tea, milk thistle and others, are natural iron-binding antioxidants. Iron can spoil nutrients within a vitamin pill. Iron should be consumed as a separate supplement. Once-weekly iron supplementation has been shown to be adequate for most people who have iron shortages. During pregnancy, a weekly iron supplement may work just as well as a daily supplement at resolving anemia. [Nutrition Hospital 13; 114, 1998] Truly anemic individuals may take iron pills daily for six weeks till a sufficient amount of red blood cells have been produced in the bone marrow. Thereafter, daily iron supplementation may not be needed.

< 125 >

Iron in Multivitamins	
Brand Name	**Amount**
Centrum Silver	0 mg
Nature Made Essential	2 mg
Mega Vita-Man-Puritan's Pride	4 mg
Centrum Select 50+	9 mg
Theragran-M—Bristol-Myers	9 mg
ABC Plus Senior-Nature's Bounty	9 mg
Daily Multi-Vitamin Mineral-Kirkland	10 mg
Ultra Mega Gold- GNC	15 mg
Multi-Vitamin Pak- Vitamin Shoppe	16 mg
Geritol Complete	18 mg
One Daily- Vitamin Shoppe	18 mg
One-A-Day Maximum	18 mg
Superior One Plus-Swanson	18 mg
Centrum Performance	18 mg
Formula 100 Puritan's Pride	18 mg
Central-Vite Rite-Aid	4-18 mg

Frankly, most multivitamin companies should warn consumers of potential problems with their products, such as iron overload. Multivitamins with iron should be accompanied by wording on labels that they are not designed for full-grown males, postmenopausal females or women who have undergone early hysterectomy.

Bottom line: Look for balanced minerals in multivitamins. Calcium and magnesium should be provided in near-equal ratios, or a little more magnesium than calcium. Calcium citrate is the best absorbable form of calcium, particularly in between meals when stomach acid levels are low. Zinc should not exceed 25 milligrams or additional copper may be needed to prevent a rise in cholesterol. Copper and iron should be consumed from the diet and be left out of vitamin pills of full-grown adults. Growing children and pregnant and lactating females

< 126 >

probably will benefit from supplemental iron. Full-grown males and postmenopausal females should guard against iron overload.

Lutein/zeaxanthin should be included in every multivitamin pill along with beta carotene.

Riboflavin (vitamin B2) is an essential B vitamin required for cell growth. Deficiencies of riboflavin can lead to skin conditions (dermatitis) and cataracts. [Metabolic & Pediatric Ophthalmology 5: 17-20, 1991] Riboflavin combines with vitamin C to produce an antioxidant enzyme called

> ### *Avoid multivitamins with excessive riboflavin (vitamin B2)*

glutathione reductase. Riboflavin in vitamin pills is what causes your urine to look yellow. However, riboflavin is a light-sensitive nutrient. [Experimental Eye Research 14: 605-609, 1992] It is easily destroyed by exposure to light. While riboflavin deficiency can lead to cataracts, excessive levels of riboflavin in the human eye, a transparent organ that is exposed to solar ultraviolet radiation, may accelerate the onset of retinal problems, floaters and cataracts. [Experentia 49: 1084-87, 1993; Inherited & Environmentally Induced Retinal Degenerations, Alan R. Liss 1989; arch Klin Exp Ophthal 194: 277, 1975; Current Eye Res 13: 505, 1994] Excessive riboflavin consumption may also lead to accelerated aging of the skin. [Free Radical Biology Med 22: 1139, 1997; J Photochem Photobiology 14: 105, 1992] Though riboflavin is an essential vitamin, and vitamin E abolishes some of its toxicity [Free Radical Biology & Medicine 24: 798-808, 1998], researchers suggest no more than 10 mg of riboflavin as a daily dosage. [Proceedings Natl Academy of Sciences 76: 3504-06, 1979] Many mega-dose vitamin pills provide excessive levels of riboflavin (25, 50, even 100 mg) which may lead to the premature loss of sight.

Beta carotene for vitamin A

Vitamin A is worthy of discussion in this book for no other reason than there is so much misplaced fear over potential liver toxicity. In recent years

< 127 >

the health authorities have issued erroneous public warnings concerning the possible overdose among adults taking vitamin A supplements. The widespread dissemination of these warnings, and their alarming tone, simply don't match the remote threat to public health. Donald R. Davis, PhD, says *"Possibly no other health hazard is cited so frequently but occurs so rarely."* [Megascorbate Therapies, Vol. 2, No. 1, Vitamin C Foundation 1997] High-dose vitamin A supplements have been available for years without one reported fatality. For comparison, aspirin tablets cause more reported deaths per year but the public is not warned away.

The first warning in 1990 suggested the ideal intake of vitamin A for the average man is about 3100-3300 International Units (IU) according to the 1989 edition of the Recommended Daily Allowances (RDAs). At that time it was estimated that 3 to 4 percent of the US population was taking 25,000 IU of vitamin A per day (7500 mcg) in food supplements and warned that this level of intake represented an overdose. [UPI Feb. 26, 1990] Out of a population of 250 million, that would mean around 7.5 million American adults were taking mega-dose vitamin A supplements. But no widespread liver toxicity was reported. From 1976 to 1987 the number of cases of vitamin A liver toxicity averaged fewer than ten cases per year. [Am J Clin Nutrition 49: 358, 1989] Recovery is spontaneous following discontinuation of supplemental vitamin A.

Vitamin A toxicity or pre-existing liver disease?

The news report conceded that vitamin A toxicity has only been shown to occur among adults who consistently consume more than 50,000 IU per day or young children who take more than 20,000 IU daily. A public health official indicated then that it wasn't vitamin A that induces liver toxicity per se but that 5000 IU to 10,000 IU per day could unmask a pre-existing liver condition.

Upon investigation, mega-dose vitamin A appears to be wrongly implicated in cases of liver toxicity when the underlying cause of the problem appears to over-consumption of alcohol, obesity, medications (tetracycline, steroids) and diabetes. [Am J Clin Nut 52: 183-202, 1990] Normally the human liver is 5-

< 128 >

15 percent fat, whereas a diabetic's liver consists of 25-35 percent fat. Modern medicine has no specific treatment for fatty liver beyond cessation of alcohol consumption and dietary changes. Yet the therapeutic use of the amino acid L-carnitine or IP6 rice bran extract may be helpful in reducing fat buildup in the liver. [Anticancer Res 19: 3695-98, 1999; Merck Manual, Sect. 1, Chp. 2]

More unjustified warnings

Then again in 2001 health authorities issued another bulletin, warning the public away from mega-dose vitamin A supplements. An Associated Press report said: *"Don't pop too many vitamin A supplements because large amounts, particularly megadoses available from health food stores, can be dangerous."* [Associated Press Jan. 10, 2001] A government advisory suggested 900 micrograms of vitamin A (~3000 IU) for men and 700 micrograms for women (~2300 IU) and no more than 3000 micrograms (10,000 IU) since excessive amounts may increase the risk of birth defects in the offspring of pregnant females. Millions of consumers scanned the labels on their multivitamin bottles and falsely believed they were taking too much vitamin A. Vitamin companies received thousands of calls from concerned consumers.

But the safe upper limit suddenly became the toxic level and the AP story mistakenly said this much vitamin A could cause serious liver disease and in pregnant females, birth defects in their offspring. The kicker to the story was the revelation that beta carotene-rich fruits and vegetables actually yield half as much vitamin A as previously thought, so most reference books are out of date. This fact would give more reason to take food supplements, not less. The potential problem of liver toxicity is exaggerated and appears to have the intent to scare the public away from vitamin supplements. After all, the National Academy of Sciences established a 5X safety factor, so it would be extremely difficult to produce liver toxicity.

< 129 >

Vitamin A liver toxicity is rare

In a study of 146 adults who took an average of 18,000 units of vitamin A palmitate over a 5-year period as treatment for inherited night blindness, none developed liver toxicity. [Am J Clin Nut 69: 656-63, 1999] A 5-year study of 116 adults, age 64-88 years, revealed dietary intake ranged from 2528 to 23,032 IU per day and supplements ranged from 0 to 47,000 IU without any reported cases of liver toxicity. [Am J Clin Nut 54: 878-83, 1991] No person has ever died from taking a vitamin A supplement.

Megavitamin tablets have occasionally induced vitamin A toxicity when taken for a long period of time. According to the Merck Manual, it takes doses of 100,000 IU per day (33,000 mcg) taken for months to induce toxicity. Beta carotene is metabolized in the body to vitamin A at a slow rate and ingestion of large amounts of beta carotene does not induce toxicity but can produce a yellowing of the skin. [Merck Manual, Section 1, Chp. 3]

Potential vitamin A toxicity is overstated

Another revelation is the admission by the National Academy of Sciences that 25 to 50 percent of young adults may not have sufficient stores of vitamin A in their liver. Healthy adults should have a four-month supply stored in their liver.

It is estimated that more than 20 percent of the population doesn't consume 70 percent of the recommended daily allowance for vitamin A. [Am J Clinical Nutrition 49: 358-71, 1989] More than 1 million Americans develop vitamin A deficiency each year. [The Nutrition Foundation, 1980] An estimated 42 to 65 percent of older Americans don't get enough vitamin A in their diet. [Nutritional Requirements in the Elderly, Geriatric Nutrition, Raven Press, 1990]

The National Academy of Sciences, teaming with the Associated Press, decided to irresponsibly issue a warning over harmless beta carotene,

< 130 >

and nearly harmless amounts of vitamin A, to protect a small number of people that are estimated to develop liver toxicity annually in the US. (While vitamin A supplements may not induce liver toxicity, there is concern that excessive vitamin A intake from foods and supplements may cause bone softening. See below.)

Vitamin A: fatty or beta carotene forms

Vitamin A is provided in its fatty form from fish, dairy and meat. For example, four ounces of beef liver provides over 50,000 IU of the fatty form of vitamin A. The human liver also slowly converts orange and yellow plant pigments, primarily beta carotene, into vitamin A. The fatty form of vitamin A in food supplements is usually provided as retinyl palmitate or retinyl acetate. The majority of the vitamin A provided in most multivitamins is in the non-toxic beta carotene form. Excess beta carotene is stored in the skin, and while it may cause a harmless yellowing of the skin (carotenemia), it does not induce liver toxicity. Yellowing of the skin from high-dose beta carotene consumption can be mistaken for jaundice, but carotenemia does not produce yellowing of the eyes which is characteristic of jaundice.

Understanding vitamin A

It's difficult to understand vitamin A dosage in supplements because it is required to be listed on labels in International Units (IU) but health authorities often issue information in other units of measure, such as micrograms (mcg) of beta carotene or micrograms of retinol. Yellow and orange plant pigments known as carotenoids convert to vitamin A in the liver when combined with a small amount of fat in the diet.

1 microgram of beta carotene equals 3.33 IU if vitamin A activity. Or put another way, 1 IU vitamin A activity = 0.3 mcg of retinol = 0.6 mcg of beta carotene = 7.2 mcg of any other pro-vitamin A carotenoids (e.g. alpha carotene).

< 131 >

Using the above figures, the safe upper limit for vitamin A is 10,000 IU or 3000 micrograms. However, if the vitamin A comes from beta carotene there is no potential for liver toxicity regardless of the dose. The newly revised RDA Academy of Sciences now recommends no more than 700 mcg (~2300 IU) of vitamin A (retinol) for females and 900 mcg (~3000 IU) for males. American adults consume between 5000-6000 IU of vitamin A from dietary sources daily. [Vital Health Statistics Series 11, No. 245, 2002]

Supplements use "daily values" rather than RDA for vitamin A, and most multivitamins provide 100 percent of the Daily Value or 5000 IU. Recently the Institute of Medicine set 10,000 IU as the safe upper limit for vitamin A.

Vitamin A fracture risk

Another challenge to sort out is the reported association between vitamin A and bone thinning (osteoporosis). A Harvard study of 70,000 postmenopausal females found those women consumed the most vitamin A, equal to about 6600 IU from foods and supplements over an 18-year period, had nearly double the risk of fractures compared to women who consumed the least amount of vitamin A. Beta carotene did not increase risk and use of supplemental estrogen appeared to reduce the risk. [J Am Med Assn 287: 47-54, 2002] Other studies do not confirm this finding. [J Am Med Assn 287: March 20, 2002]

At intakes not far beyond the Recommended Daily Allowance, vitamin A from food or supplements appears to affect mineral density of bone in the elderly. [J Bone Mineral Res 17: 1349-58, 2002] Healthy Americans don't need to be concerned about vitamin A deficiency since the diet provides 5000-6000 IU.

The finding that high vitamin A intake from foods or supplements may increase the risk of bone fracture is not new. Vitamin A is antagonistic to vitamin D which is required for calcium absorption and bone renewal. [J Nutrition 115: 929-35, 1985] The highest incidence of osteoporosis

< 132 >

is found in northern Europe where vitamin D production from sunlight exposure is limited and vitamin A intake is high. In humans, very high doses (30,000 IU+) of vitamin A may decrease serum calcium levels by interfering with vitamin D's role in enhancing the intestinal absorption of calcium. [J Bone Mineral Res 16: 1899-905, 2001] The answer to this problem is to avoid high-dose vitamin A and to balance vitamin A intake with vitamin D.

Vitamin A and birth defects

Vitamin A is essential for normal reproduction and childhood development. Doses of the fatty form of vitamin A exceeding 10,000 IU per day have been reported in a single study to increase the risk of birth defects. There is no observed risk from beta carotene. [Reproductive Toxicology 12: 75-88, 1998] The current recommendations for vitamin A intake during pregnancy are 800 retinol equivalents per day which is equal to 2700 IU or 4800 micrograms of beta carotene. A study conducted by the National Institutes of Health found that 8000 IU to 10,000 IU doses of vitamin A taken during pregnancy did not increase the risk of birth defects (it is rare for women to consume more than 10,000 IU of vitamin A from foods and supplements). [Am J Obstet Gynecol 177: 31-6, 1997]

Who needs more vitamin A?

The human body requires vitamin A for optimal function of the immune system, for night vision, for mucus production and for maintenance of tissues that line the internal and external surfaces of the body (epithelium).

Low-fat diets, diabetes, liver disease, infection and diarrheal diseases may impair conversion of beta carotene to vitamin A in the liver. [Nutrition Research 15: 1613-21, 1995]

< 133 >

There is an increased need for vitamin A surrounding bouts of infection. [Ann Rev Nutrition 21: 167-92, 2001] Infectious disease can decrease intake, absorption and excretion of vitamin A. [Annual Rev Nut 21: 167-92, 2001] Low levels of vitamin A are associated with greater risk for cervical cancer caused by the human papilloma virus. [Nutrition Cancer 34: 229-34, 1999] People with chronic viral infections, measles or tuberculosis may require more vitamin A. [Clin Diag Lab Immunol 9: 616-21, 2002; Proc Nut Soc 58: 719-27, 1999]

Women are advised to avoid overdosage of vitamin A from supplements because of the risk for birth defects, but pregnant females have increased demand for vitamin A to ensure the proper growth and development of their offspring. Pregnancy typically reduces circulating vitamin A levels by 25 percent. A study of American women who belonged to minority groups found 26 to 29 percent exhibited marginal vitamin A levels. Low birth weight is associated with low vitamin A levels in mothers. [Nutrition Research 15: 1263-76, 1995]

In a small study, 11 healthy men were given beta carotene supplements with a fatty meal which is required for the conversion of beta carotene to vitamin A in the liver. But only 6 of the 11 exhibited a measurable rise in circulating vitamin A levels, which means conversion of beta carotene to vitamin A can be surprisingly low and prolonged in some individuals. [Am J Clin Nut 75: 900-07, 2002; Nutrition Reviews 60: 104-10, 2002] This report is significant given that about 50 percent of dietary vitamin A is obtained from beta carotene and 50 percent in fatty form from meat, fish and dairy products.

In conditions where dietary intake of the fatty form of vitamin A is insufficient and in states of chronic or prolonged infection, supplementation with less than 5000 IU is suggested. [Seminars Perinatology 21: 135-42, 1997] Of interest, vegetarian diets that only acquire vitamin A from carotenoids in plant foods do not result in low circulating levels of vitamin A which is a measure of stored vitamin A in the liver. [Int J Vitam Nut Res 60: 58-66, 1990]

< 134 >

Beta carotene pills superior to foods

Beta carotene pills may be superior to beta carotene in foods. While Americans are frequently advised to obtain essential nutrients from foods, a study conducted among women in an undeveloped country showed that a beta carotene pill improved vitamin A status better than foods. [The Lancet 346: 75, 1995] This study reveals that beta carotene in pill form can often improve vitamin A status better than dark-green leafy vegetables. Furthermore, a recent

> **Beta carotene in pills is superior to beta carotene in foods**

report issued from the National Academies of Sciences shows it takes twice as much plant foods such as carrots, broccoli and sweet potatoes, as previously believed to produce a given amount of vitamin A. [Natl Acad Sci, Jan, 9, 2001] A carrot provides plenty of fiber which impedes beta carotene absorption whereas a beta carotene pill contains no fiber to interfere with absorption.

Beta carotene is not only beneficial because it produces vitamin A. Studies indicate beta carotene helps to keep cholesterol particles from oxidizing (hardening). [Free Radical Biology Med 17: 537-44, 1994]

Vitamin A: brand analysis

The amount of vitamin A provided in multivitamins varies widely and the percentage of the fatty form of vitamin A (retinyl palmitate or acetate) or from beta carotene also varies. Brands of multivitamins appear to be oblivious to the fact that the American diet provides a sufficient amount of vitamin A and that further provision of the fatty form of vitamin A may interfere with vitamin D absorption which in turn may impair bone health. Here is a selected group of brand-name multivitamins and their vitamin A analysis:

< 135 >

Brand of multivitamin	Fatty form Vitamin A	Vitamin A from beta carotene
Life Extension	5000 IU acetate	5000 IU
Centrum Select 50	3000 IU	6000 IU
Centrum Silver	4000 IU	1000 IU
Century Formula	5000 IU acetate	—
Daily One Caps - Twinlab	—	5000 IU
Daily 2 Multiple Nature's Way	7425 IU palmitate	15,075 IU
Forward Plus-Whitaker	5000 IU palmitate	15,000 IU
Geritol Complete	—	7250 IU
Iron Free VM-75-Solgar	7500 IU palmitate	7500 IU
Mega Vita-Min-Puritan Pride	8000 IU	—
Multi Ultra Mega Gold GNC	5000 IU acetate	15,000 IU
One-A-Day Men's	3010 IU	490 IU
Perfect Multi-Purity	—	10,000 IU
Prime Years-Schiff	—	5000 IU
Rite-Aid Central-Vite	2500 IU	2500 IU
Theragran M Advanced	4000 IU ?	1000 IU
Whole Source-Rite Aid	2550 IU acetate	4950 IU
Amount of vitamin A provided by the typical American diet: 5000 IU		
Amount of vitamin A needed in food supplements: 0		
Amount of vitamin A required to produce long-term side effects: 25,000 IU		
Beta carotene is converted to vitamin A in the liver and excesses are stored in the skin, which means beta carotene exhibits no liver toxicity (liver buildup).		

< 136 >

Bottom line: Multivitamins should provide vitamin A for well-nourished populations solely in the beta carotene form. Since there is no toxicity from beta carotene, no limit is suggested though there may be some competition for absorption between carotenoids (beta carotene and lutein/zeaxanthin), so balanced carotenoids are recommended. Persons with chronic infections or other special circumstances such as night blindness should obtain vitamin A in its fatty form (retinyl acetate or palmitate).

< 137 >

Vitamin Truth #11
Use Multivitamins that
Aid Absorption

About 13 percent less digestive juice is produced for every decade of life. [Geriatric Nutrition, Raven Press, 1990] This means at age 50 you may have lost over 30 percent of your ability to produce digestive juice. That's why by middle age, many adults simply have trouble digesting foods and vitamin pills.

The Problem of Absorption		
Percentage of mature adults with nutritional deficiencies before and after taking vitamin supplements.		
	Before taking vitamin pills	**After taking vitamin pills**
Vitamin B1-Thiamin	13-40%	0-6%
Vitamin B2-Riboflavin	3-42%	0%
Vitamin B3-Niacin	0-33%	0-33%
Vitamin B6-Pyridoxine	19-56%	2-29%
Folic acid	14-43%	0-13%
Vitamin B12	4-43%	0-18%
Source: Nutritional Requirements of the elderly, W.R. Bidlack, in Geriatric Nutrition, Raven Press, New York, 1990.		

In some cases, rock-hard vitamin tablets, which are produced by compression, pass right through the digestive tract. Stories abound of older adults who notice their vitamin tablets go through their digestive system intact and end up in the toilet bowl. In one study 4 of 11 brands of multivitamin tablets failed to disintegrate even when exposed to simulated stomach acid conditions. [J Renal Nutrition 9: 78-83, 1999] A study of folic acid supplements found a third of the brands of multivitamins studied did not dissolve in a timely fashion. To meet USP dissolution requirements at least 75 percent of the labeled amount should be released in 1 hour. [J Am Pharm Assn NS37: 397-400, 1997]

< 138 >

One study showed capsules superior to tablets by 36 percent. [J Pharm Sci 68: 104-06, 1979] An estimated 30 to 50 percent of adults may not produce enough digestive juice to properly absorb vitamins. Vitamin tablets continue to be made that do not meet USP dissolution standards. No USP dissolution standards are required for gelatin capsules since it is known they break down more readily. Well-designed vitamin pills will often include plant enzymes like bromelain (from pineapple) and papain (from papaya) and betaine to improve nutrient absorption.

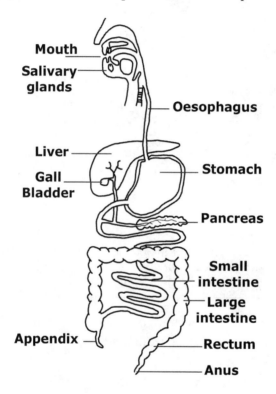

Factors involved in utilization of vitamins and minerals
A. Intake. B. Dissolution or breakdown of vitamin pills. C. Absorption dependent upon stomach acid and enzymes. D. Transport. Fatty nutrients like vitamin E and lutein are carried on cholesterol particles to tissues F. Storage. Fatty nutrients like vitamin A and D are stored in the liver, vitamin E in adipose (fatty) tissue for future use.

< 139 >

Vitamin Truth #12
Skip Adding an Aspirin To Your Multivitamin Regimen

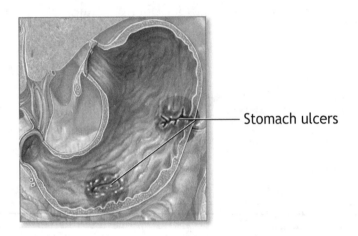

🍂A.D.A.M.

Even low-dose coated aspirin tablets can produce bleeding stomach ulcers. Many of the health benefits of aspirin can be obtained by taking a good multivitamin.

Aspirin thins the blood and inhibits blood clots. Studies show adults who take a daily aspirin tablet reduce their risk of a heart attack and stroke. [Archives Internal Med 154: 2649-57, 1994] Others take aspirin for pain relief. But consumers are not told that aspirin increases the risk of a hemorrhagic stroke and bleeding at the back of the eyes (retina). [Survey of Ophthalmology 37: 149, 1992] Aspirin depletes the body of folic acid, iron, potassium, sodium and vitamin C. [Drug Nutrient Depletion Handbook 2nd Ed, 2001] Aspirin also impairs the absorption of vitamin C by 70 percent. [Biochemical Pharmacology 31: 4035-38, 1982] Aspirin and other non-steroidal anti-inflammatory drugs are now responsible for 15 percent of the gastric ulcers and coated aspirin tablets don't completely eliminate this potential problem. Even low-dose

< 140 >

coated aspirin pills can cause a bleeding stomach ulcer. [Am J Gastroent 97: 2215-19, 2002] So many millions of Americans have to take acid-suppressant drugs to prevent heartburn, particularly after meals. Aspirin users are ten times more likely to be taking acid-blockers (Pepcid, Zantac, Prilosec, Nexium). [Postgraduate Medicine 76: 734-35, 2000] Many people are unaware that aspirin may

Aspirin depletes the body of essential nutrients

not always work. Many people have inborn or developed resistance to aspirin and confer no protection from cardiovascular mortality. [Ann Pharm 36: 1620, 2002]

We lose about a spoon full of blood every time we ingest an aspirin tablet. Blood in the stool can then cause a positive stool test and result in adults having to undergo needless diagnostic procedures to search for non-existent colon cancer.

Fortunately there are alternatives to aspirin. The man who introduced one-a-day aspirin to prevent heart attacks says nature provides compounds that work even better. Bioflavonoids, plant pigments obtained from citrus rind, grapes and berries are better blood-thinners than aspirin. Quercetin is a widely studied bioflavonoid found naturally in onions which exhibits both pain relieving and blood thinning properties. [Cardiology World News May-June 1996]

< 141 >

Vitamin Truth #13
Some Synthetic Vitamins Are Perfectly Acceptable

Unfortunately, unwitting consumers are often duped by unfounded claims that synthetic vitamins are undesirable and that certain brands of vitamins are entirely natural. Many vitamins, like vitamin C and all the B vitamins, must be made synthetically, since there is no economical way to extract sufficient amounts from foods. Coenzyme Q10 and alpha lipoic acid are examples of non-vitamin nutrients that are synthetically produced. So it's easy to see how consumers can become confused over the issue of natural vs. synthetic vitamins.

Another sales pitch often heard is that food-based vitamins are superior. Food-based vitamins, if they were to be provided in the doses needed for optimal health, would cost a small fortune. Food-based vitamin pills can only provide trivial amounts of nutrients, not enough to reach optimal health goals. For example, with advancing age there is a common problem in absorbing food-bound vitamin B12, but not B12 from supplements. [J Am Geriatrics Society 50: 1789, 2002] A carrot provides about 10,000 units of vitamin A activity from beta carotene, but little of it is absorbed due to the high fiber content. Food supplements will provide more beta carotene than beta-carotene-rich foods.

< 142 >

Vitamin Truth #14
Make Sure What's on the Label Is in the Bottle

Recent studies have revealed that in some instances nutritional supplements do not provide the level of nutrients printed on the label. People inside the food supplement industry indicate some companies try to compete by skimping on ingredients, hoping they won't get caught. In some instances, tests have shown the labels don't match the levels of nutrients provided in the product, but the companies often respond by saying there must have been some oversight in that particular batch. How can consumers be assured they are getting their money's worth when it comes to vitamins? One way is to only purchase from reputable companies. Another is to ask for written certification. Some companies will provide a certificate of analysis upon request. Inside tip: buy freshly-made vitamins. Reputable manufacturers customarily pack 10 to 15 percent more nutrients inside each pill than the stated dosage on the label in order to make up for small losses of nutrients during prolonged shelf storage. You may get more than you paid for if you buy freshly-made products. The freshest product would ideally be shipped directly from manufacturer to consumer rather than remain in storage warehouses or retail shelves for months prior to purchase.

< 143 >

Vitamin Truth #15
How Many Pills Does It Take To Get That Much Nutrition?

It's difficult to compare brands of vitamins because many times products appear to provide about the same amount of nutrients but the consumer never notices how many pills have to be taken each day to get that much supplemental nutrition. One product on the market requires consumers to take 12 pills per day. Another potent multivitamin only requires six pills per day, but in order to make the product appear price-competitive, the bottle provides only a 10-day supply so consumers have to purchase three bottles per month. Often times the consumer doesn't realize the difference till after they have purchased the product and broken the seal on the cap and then they are reluctant to return the product.

Pay careful attention to the suggested number of pills you have to take to obtain the dosages printed on the label. A good multivitamin, with dosages of nutrients that provide optimal health benefits, will likely require 3-6 capsules per day, which is fewer pills than taking every nutrient individually.

< 144 >

Vitamin Truth #16
Multivitamins Can and Should
Include Phytonutrients

Phytonutrients are derived from plants. Herbs and spices are well known for their medicinal properties and are often added to progressive multivitamin formulas. Sometimes these exotic herbs and spices are added to multivitamins at the expense of essential vitamins and minerals. Consumers should look for multivitamin products that are centered around essential nutrients.

However, with 80 percent or more of the the American diet comprised of processed foods, the addition of some herbs and spices would likely mimic intake from a plant-food based diet. The health benefits of plant extracts from green tea, ginger, ginseng, milk thistle, ginkgo biloba, turmeric, rosemary, soy, spirulina, aloe vera, and other herbs and spices are now being widely reported. [J Nutrition 13: 3034S, 2001; Am J Clin Nut 70: 491S, 1999] If there is room for some of these powerful antioxidants and nutrients in your multivitamin pill, they are certainly desirable.

In one study, green tea extract was found to exhibit antioxidant power 32 times that of vitamin E. This means just 10 mg of green tea is equal to 320 units of vitamin E in antioxidant protection (though green tea doesn't replace vitamin E in the antioxidant defense system). Plant-based nutrients make handsome additions to any multivitamin.

There is one obscure but important phytonutrient worth mentioning. There is a flurry of research surrounding an antioxidant found in blueberries, plums, pineapples, corn, pine bark, rice bran, bee hive propolis, Ginkbo biloba and the herb Artemisia. It is ferulic acid. Here is what researchers are discovering about ferulic acid. It is a strong antioxidant particularly in nervous tissues like the brain, making it a potential agent for treatment of brain diseases. [J Nutr Biochem 13: 273-

< 145 >

81, 2002] In extremely high experimental doses, equivalent to 1000 mg in a human, ferulic acid in animals prevented any adverse effects in the brain from beta amyloid peptide, the protein that is believed to impair memory in Alzheimer's disease. [Br J Pharm 133: 89-96, 2001]

One important phytonutrient is ferulic acid

It is a natural COX-2 inhibitor, or anti-inflammatory agent on the order of similar inflammation-fighting drugs. [Bioorganic Med Chem 10: 1189-96, 2002] In rice bran, ferulic acid is found within gamma oryzanol, a strong cholesterol-lowering agent. [J Food Sci Tech 30: 249-52, 1993] Relatively low doses have been demonstrated to reduce blood pressure in animals. [Am J Hypertension 15: 351-57, 2002] Ferulic acid inhibits the growth of breast and colon cancer cells. [Cancer Epid Biomark Prev 9: 1163-70, 2000] Ferulic acid absorbs potentially harmful solar ultraviolet radiation, making it a natural sun screen to protect the skin and eyes from aging. [Int J Pharm 199: 39-47, 2000] Ferulic acid appears to raise HDL "good" cholesterol. [Lipids 35: 427-35, 2000] Ferulic acid has a natural tranquilizing effect different from drugs. [Arzneimittleforschung 43: 715-21, 1993] Maybe ferulic acid will soon make the list of plant nutrients (phytonutrients) added to multivitamins. Some consumers look suspiciously upon these herbs and spices when added to vitamin preparations but don't think twice about them in foods.

< 146 >

Vitamin Truth #17
Cheap Vitamins Will Cost
You a Fortune

An estimated $2.710 billion of multivitamins are sold annually in the US. [Nutrition Business Journal] A Consumer Reports survey shows that many Americans spend as little as $3 per month, or about 10 cents per day, on vitamin supplements. [Consumer Reports 59: 561-69, 1994] <u>To obtain the dosages of nutrients outlined in scientific studies that prevent or delay the onset of heart attacks, cancer, cataracts and other health problems, consumers will need to spend a dollar or more per day for a multivitamin.</u> That's a small price to pay for the best health insurance.

There is no question that many American consumers are resistant when it comes to spending money on vitamins, believing their health plan or Medicare should pay for them. Many Americans spend more money on pet food than they do on health maintenance.

Expenditure	Annual amount spent	Spent per day
Auto repair	$366	$1.00
Alcohol	$222	$0.61
Prescription drugs	$216	$0.59
Tobacco	$170	$0.47
Vitamins	$ 80	$0.22
US Dept. of Commerce Bureau Economic Analyses 1997		

Don't jeopardize your health with cheap multivitamins that sell you short. The most expensive vitamin is the cheapest one you can buy.

On an average day, Americans spend $434 million on toys, $24.6 million on donuts, $21.9 million on cosmetics, $10.4 million on potato chips,

< 147 >

$8.5 million on dog food, $5.8 million on cat food, $5.5 million on bird food and $3.7 million on vitamin pills.

On an average day, Americans swallow:
80 million aspirin tablets
13 million tranquilizers
13 million sleeping pills

Americans spend annually, $4000 per person on health insurance, diagnosis and treatment of disease, $1000 in additional out-of-pocket health care expenses, and only about $80 a year on vitamins.

Vitamin and Supplement Survey	
How often do you take vitamins and mineral supplements:	
Daily	49%
Sometimes	23%
Weekly	7%
Monthly	3%
Never	18%
Source: American Dietetic Assn Trends 2000 Survey	

8 in 10 Americans do not consume the recommended 5 servings of fresh fruits and vegetables daily and should be taking multivitamins.

< 148 >

Summary

Don't wait till you have a health problem before you consider taking multivitamins. A National Health Interview Survey conducted in 1992 found only 24 percent of Americans use vitamins of any kind on a daily basis, but 70 percent of men age 43-54 years with heart disease took a multivitamin. [J Nutrition 128: 2355-62, 1998]

One false assumption is that people don't need antioxidant supplement until they become unhealthy. But the Journal of the American Medical Association admits the destructive process of oxidation is involved in virtually every disease. [J Am Med Assn 271: 1148-49, 1994] Supplemental anti-rusting agents known as antioxidants are beneficial in delaying premature aging and in preventing disease.

Multivitamins should be balanced, potent and complete

A modern multivitamin ought to provide an array of essential nutrients which includes the complete family of B vitamins, all of the essential minerals and other important non-vitamin nutrients such as lutein, chromium, coenzyme Q10 and sources of sulfur (alpha lipoic acid, N-acetyl cysteine, taurine). Look for brands that *"cover the bases"* and provide all the elements of *"The Antioxidant Tree"* rather than just a few antioxidants. There are limits—your multivitamin cannot provide you with mega-doses of all the minerals and other antioxidants suggested in scientific reports. You would have to consume a *"horse-sized"* pill to get everything from a multivitamin pill. For example, all the calcium and magnesium your body needs is just too bulky to fit into a multivitamin pill. So look for brands that provide a minimum of important nutrients, like 200 units of vitamin E with accompanying mixed tocopherols and tocotrienols, 500 mg of vitamin C, an ample amount of bioflavonoids (representing 70 percent or more of the vitamin C), over 150 mcg. of

< 149 >

selenium, 800 mcg of folic acid, plus potent amounts of vitamin B12 (300 mcg. or more).

<u>Look for brands that are balanced</u>: The full family of vitamin E tocopherols and tocotrienols; no more than 15-25 mg of zinc with balanced copper from the diet; supplemental magnesium should be equal to or exceed levels of calcium; beta carotene and lutein/zeaxanthin should be provided in near-equal doses (6 mg); and high doses of beta carotene should be avoided so as not to overwhelm lutein and impair its absorption.

<u>Look for brands that include</u> a full 6 mg of lutein/zeaxanthin, coenzyme Q10, chromium and sources of sulfur (taurine, lipoic acid, MSM and glutathione).

<u>Look for brands that don't overdose on certain nutrients</u>. One of the major failings of multivitamin manufacturers is their inability to factor dietary intake against daily nutritional needs. The American diet provide sufficient amounts of vitamin A, calcium and iron, nutrients that do not need to be supplemented. Mature adults and non-menstruating females should avoid supplements that provide iron. Riboflavin should not exceed 10 mg per day. High doses of zinc (more than 25 mg) should be avoided to prevent a rise in cholesterol.

<u>Look for brands that provide the potent and highly absorbable forms of nutrients</u>, such as natural-source vitamin E (d-alpha tocopherol) rather than synthetic vitamin E (dl-alpha tocopherol); organic selenium yeast (SelenoExcel™) rather than inorganic forms (sodium selenate or selenite); easy-to-absorb vitamin B12 (methylcobalamin rather than cyanocobalamin) and calcium citrate rather than calcium carbonate.

< 150 >

< 151 >

How To Read a
Food Supplement Label

EXAMPLE

Supplement Facts
Serving Size 1 tablet

Amount Per Serving	% Daily Value
Vitamin A 5000 IU	
50% as beta carotene	100% (1)
Vitamin C 250 mg	417% (2)
Vitamin D 400 IU	100% (3)
Vitamin E dl-Alpha tocopherol 200 IU	667% (4)
Thiamin 25 mg	1665% (5)
Riboflavin 25 mg	1470% (6)
Niacin 20 mg	100% (7)
Vitamin B6 5 mg	250% (8)
Folic Acid 0.4 mg	100% (9)
Vitamin B12 6 mcg cyanocobalamin	100% (10)
Biotin 150 mcg	50%
Pantothenic acid 10 mg	100%
Calium carbonate 100 mg	10% (11)
Iron 18 mg	100% (12)
Iodine 150 mcg	100%
Selenium 35 mcg selenate	50% (13)
Magnesium 50 mg	12.5% (14)
Zinc oxide 15 mg	100% (15)
Copper 2 mg	100% (16)
Boron 150 mcg	*
Lutein/zeaxanthin 250 mcg	* (17)
Lycopene 3 mg	* (18)

* Daily Value not established

(19) **Ingredients:** FD&C Red 40 Lake; gelatin; magnesium stearate

< 152 >

Comment number	Topic	Comment
1	Vitamin A 5000 IU 50% as beta carotene	Should be 100% beta carotene in USA; Americans consume 5000 IU vitamin A from the diet
2	Vitamin C 250 mg	Doesn't indicate type of vitamin C; Dosage not enough for optimal health
3	Vitamin D 400 IU	Gives false impression 100% is enough; 800 IU needed to prevent fractures
4	Vitamin E dl-alpha tocopherol 200 IU	dl designates synthetic vitamin E; natural source vitamin E preferred
5	Thiamin 25 mg	Gives false impression of overdose
6	Riboflavin 25 mg	Excessive; limit to 10 mg; photosensitizing vitamin; excess may induce eye and skin troubles
7	Vitamin B6 5 mg	Gives false impression of excessive dose
8	Folic acid 0.4 mg	Not enough according to latest science; 800 mcg now recommended
9	Vitamin B12 6 mcg cyanocobalamin	Gives false impression 100% is enough; methylcobalamin is better absorbed
10	Calcium carbonate 100 mg	Bulky mineral; multi's cannot provide 100%; citrate form is better absorbed
11	Iron 18 mg	Not recommended for grown males, postmenopausal females
12	Selenium 35 mcg selenate	Inorganic form; not desirable; dosage is weak

< 153 >

Comment number	Topic	Comment
13	Magnesium 50 mg	Not enough to prevent sudden-heart spasm; not balanced with calcium
14	Zinc oxide 15 mg	Oxides are poorly absorbed
15	Copper 2 mg	1 mg copper for 10 mg zinc ratio
16	Boron 150 mcg	Need 3000 mcg; impotent dosage
17	Lutein/ zeaxanthin 250 mcg	Weak dose; 6000 mcg needed for eye health
18	Lycopene 3 mg	Diet provides adequate amounts (tomato source 20 mg); foods are more economical
19	Ingredients	Undesirable food coloring added; other ingredients acceptable

< 154 >

Master Guide to Nutrient Intake

Nutrient	Typical Dietary Intake	New Dietary Ref. Intake	Amt for Optimal Health to be Obtained from Supplements	Tolerable Upper Limit Actually Safe Upper Limit	No Observed Adverse Effect Level	Lowest Observed Adverse Effect Level
CAROTENOIDS						
Beta carotene	7500 IU (2496 mcg)	--	10,000 IU+	25,000 mcg	None est.	
Lutein/ zeaxanthin	2314 mcg (low of 1768 in mid-age females)	None est.	6000 mcg	None est.	--	--
Lycopene	6296 mcg (up to 12964 mcg in males)	None est.	0	None est.	--	--
VITAMINS						
Vitamin A	6542 IU	2700 IU (900 mcg) males) 2100 IU (700 mcg) females	0	10,000 IU (3000 mcg)	21,600 IU (6500 mcg)	
Vitamin B1 thiamin	1.7 mg	1.2 mg	Unknown supplement for alcoholics	50 mg	None est.	
Vitamin B2 riboflavin	1.9 mg		No more than 10 mg	10 mg*		
Vitamin B3 niacin	24.1 mg	16 mg	Unknown	35 mg	1500 mg nicotina-mide	3000 mg nicotina-mide
Vitamin B5 panto-thenic acid	ww	5 mg	Unknown	None est.	None est.	
Vitamin B6 pyridoxine	1.9 mg	1.7 mg	25-50 mg	100 mg	200 mg	--
Vitamin B9 folic acid	291 mcg	400 mcg	800+ mcg	1000 mcg	--	--
Vitamin B12 cobalamin	5.2 mcg	2.4 mcg	300-1000 mcg	None est.	--	--

< 155 >

Nutrient	Typical Dietary Intake	New Dietary Ref. Intake	Amt for Optimal Health to be Obtained from Supplements	Tolerable Upper Limit Actually Safe Upper Limit	No Observed Adverse Effect Level	Lowest Observed Adverse Effect Level
VITAMINS						
Biotin		300 mcg?		None est.	2500 mcg	None est.
Choline		550 mg	Bulky; need from diet	3500 mg	--	--
Vitamin C	109 mg	90 mg	300-2000 mg	2000+ mg	None est.	--
Vitamin D	4.9 mcg (196 IU)	600 IU (15 mcg)	800+ IU (20 mcg)	2000 IU (50 mcg)	40,000 IU*	--
Vitamin E	9.6 mg	15 mg	200-300 IU	1000 mg 1200 IU	None est.	--
MINERALS						
Calcium	782 mg (1208 high males)	1300 mg 1200-1500 mg	0 to 600 mg	2000 mg 2500 mg		2000 mg
Magnesium	309 mg (235 mg low)	420 mg	200-400 mg	350 mg (supplements only)	--	--
Potassium Sodium intake 3351-4000 mg/day	2993 mg		500-1000 mg	None est	--	--
Iron	15.6 mg	18.0 mg	0	45 mg	65 mg	100 mg
Manganese	1.0-9.0 mg	2.3 mg males 1.8 mg females	Unknown	11 mg	10 mg	None est.
Zinc	12.2. mg	11 mg	15-25 mg	40 mg	30 mg	60 mg
Copper	1400 mcg	900 mcg	0	10000 mcg	9000 mcg	None est.
Boron	2-3 mg	None est.	3-10 mg	20 mg	--	--
Chromium	50 mcg	35 mcg	200 mcg	None est.	1000 mcg	None est.
Iodine		150 mcg		1100 mcg	1000 mcg	None est.
Selenium	80 mcg	55 mcg	150-200 mcg	400 mcg	200 mcg	910 mcg

Dietary intake: Mean Intake per day, U.S. 1988-94, both sexes, age 50-59
Vital and Health Statistics, Dietary Intake of Macronutrients, 1988-94, Series 11, No. 245, 2002

< 156 >

Questions and Answers about Multivitamins

Question: What makes urine turn yellow when taking multivitamins?
Answer: Riboflavin (vitamin B2) is usually the reason for the yellow appearance of urine when taking vitamin supplements.

Question: What causes brown specks to occur in vitamin pills?
Answer: B vitamins are the most vulnerable to spoilage in multivitamins. B vitamins are easily (oxidized) by light, heat and moisture, which is why vitamins come in dark bottles and consumers are advised to store them in dark, dry areas. The appearance of brown specks in a vitamin pill is an indication the B vitamins have begun to spoil.

Question: Why am I nauseated after taking multivitamins?
Answer: Multivitamins may provide the nutritional equivalent of 25 pounds of food. Enzymes and stomach acid must be secreted to digest this amount of nutrients. Otherwise nutrients will ferment rather than digest and air and gas will result. It is important to take multivitamin pills with a meal since chewing and food activate the necessary enzymes and acids to properly break down and assimilate vitamins and minerals. Persistent problems may mean supplemental enzymes or hydrochloric acid may be needed (don't take hydrochloric acid supplements if you can't tolerate acidic foods or you have a stomach ulcer).

Question: Can I double up and take twice the amount of the dime-a-day vitamins?
Answer: Doubling-up on cheap vitamins may save money, but you will then be taking too much zinc and possibly other nutrients. It's best to take a well-designed vitamin formula.

< 157 >

Question: Why don't multivitamins provide enough calcium and magnesium?

Answer: Calcium and magnesium are bulky minerals that cannot be supplied in adequate amounts in multivitamin pills without taking 8-12 pills a day. It's best to take a separate mineral formula.

Question: Will a multivitamin interfere with my medications?

Answer: This is a misdirected question. Vitamins and minerals are essential for health, synthetically produced drugs are not. In many instances adults would not require medications if they were taking a well designed multivitamin. Many medications deplete the body of essential nutrients and supplements are required.

< 158 >

Drug	Nutrients depleted
Ace inhibitors (Enalapirl, Vasotec)	Zinc
Acetaminophen (Tylenol)	Glutathione
Acid blockers (Prilosec, Zantac, Pepcid, Nexium)	Vitamin B12, folic acid, vitamin D, zinc
Antidepressants (Elavil, Sinequan)	Vitamin B2, coenzyme Q10
Anti-inflammatory Cox-2 inhibitors (Celebrex)	Folic acid
Aspirin	Folic acid, potassium, sodium, vitamin C, iron
Beta blocker (Timolol, Timoptic)	Coenzyme Q10
Calcium blocker (Atenolol, Tenormin)	Coenzyme Q10
Digitalis (Digoxin, Lanoxin)	Vitamin B1, calcium, magnesium, phosphorus
Estrogen (Premarin)	Vitamin B6, magnesium
Hydrocodone (Vicodin)	Glutathione
Ibuprofen	Folic acid
Statin cholesterol-lowering drugs (Lipitor, Zocor, Lovastatin, Pravachol, Advicor)	Coenzyme Q10
Steroids (cortisone, prednisone)	Calcium, magnesium, potassium, selenium, vitamin C, vitamin D, zinc
Oral contraceptives	Magnesium, vitamin B2, vitamin B6, vitamin C

Source: Drug-Induced Nutrient Depletion Handbook, 2nd edition, 2001

Question: What about fillers and excipients in vitamin pills?
Answer: Beginning in 1999 food supplement manufacturers were required to list on labels all of the incidental ingredients in their products. Under "other ingredients" consumers will find additives required to bind tablets together, coatings for tablets, lubricants to help make powder flow, colorings and fillers. Examples of inert additives are titanium dioxide

< 159 >

and silicon dioxide (silica). Other natural additives are cellulose, starches and gums. Undesirable additives include lactose, corn starch, sucrose, FD & C dyes and hydrogenated vegetable oils. The primary problem with additives is in tablets, not capsules. Too often vitamin companies make a big issue over trivial additives in vitamin pills while these same companies haven't done their homework and offer multivitamins that are typically impotent, unbalanced and incomplete.

Question: What single nutrient is not provided in multivitamins that most of the population is deficient in and needs to take supplements?
Answer: Better than 8 in 10 Americans are deficient in omega-3 oils, essential for human health. Omega-3 oils, provided as fish oil or flaxseed oil, are needed for the proper functioning of the immune and nervous system, to reduce inflammation, and the production of hormones. A well designed multivitamin and a bottle of fish or flaxseed oil will meet 99 percent of the essential nutrient needs to maintain health.

Question: What can I do if I have difficulty swallowing vitamin pills?
Answer: About 20 percent of the public can't swallow pills very well. Sometimes this is caused by dry mouth. Two-piece capsules can be opened and the powder placed in a cold drink like tomato juice. A drink that will mask the sour flavor of vitamins is needed. Some people find they can swallow pills better if they bend over and let the pills rise to the roof of their mouth before downing them. Don't ever take gelatin capsules with hot liquids or it may dissolve the gelatin before it reaches the stomach.

Question: Are food-based vitamins superior to synthetic vitamins?
Answer: Food-based vitamins are derived from foods but are very costly on a milligram basis. There simply is no economical way to obtain the therapeutic and preventive doses of vitamins from foods. Just 500 milligrams of vitamin C would cost many dollars per day if derived from foods. Synthetic vitamins are proven to be active in all clinical studies and make vitamin supplements affordable to all.

< 160 >

Examples of nutrients in food supplements that are superior to those found in foods		
Folic acid	Some people genetically cannot absorb food-bound folic acid very well	Food-bound folic acid not as bioavailable as in vitamin pills
Beta carotene	Fiber content of carrots, sweet potatoes, yams limits absorption of beta carotene	Beta carotene from food supplements is better absorbed
Vitamin B12	As little as 1% absorbed from diet	Absorption of mega-dose methylcobalamin form of vitamin B12 superior to that in foods
Vitamin C	Foods provide small amounts of vitamin C (orange = 60 mg)	Food supplements can provide enough vitamin C to prevent disease and prolong life (300 mg+)
Vitamin D	Winter in northern latitudes and being homebound impairs natural vitamin D production in the skin from sun exposure	Dietary sources of vitamin D cannot make up for lack of sun exposure in winter or among home bound individuals
Calcium	Calcium in foods requires stomach acid for absorption; ~30% of older adults do not produce sufficient amounts of stomach acid	Calcium citrate requires no stomach acid for absorption
Zinc	Small amounts absorbed from foods	Zinc in food supplements more bioavailable

Question: What about liquid vitamins and colloidal minerals?
Answer: Vitamins and minerals in liquid form may be better absorbed which is the chief benefit promoted by manufacturers of these products. For example, magnesium in bottled water is absorbed about 30 to 40 percent better than in plant foods. Liquid vitamins do have a limited shelf life and since B vitamins are not very tasty, flavoring usually needs to be added to mask the undesirable taste. Colloidal minerals are frequently touted for being better absorbed, but please refer to the

< 161 >

section below regarding the false assumption that enhanced mineral absorption is always beneficial. Colloidal minerals are obtained from humic shale and offer an array of 77 minerals, only 17 which are the primary essential minerals. Shale may contain heavy metals such as mercury, lead, cadmium, silver and gold which are undesirable. While plant foods provide a small amount of these heavy metals, their intentional consumption is questionable.

Question: Should I get a blood test to determine if I am deficient in any nutrients?
Answer: Blood tests only provide information on recent history and intake of nutrients. Furthermore, certain blood tests are notoriously inaccurate, such as serum blood levels of zinc and magnesium. Additionally, high blood levels do not indicate tissue levels of nutrients. Finally, high blood levels may provide a false impression of adequacy. For example, a high calcium level in the blood serum may mean the body is excreting or losing this mineral from the bones at an accelerated rate. The best way to eliminate deficiencies is to eat a diet rich in plant foods and take a well designed multivitamin, so shortages never occur.

Question: What are the common symptoms of nutrient deficiencies?
Answer: While symptoms may not be the most accurate way of determining nutritional deficiencies, they may provide a clue as to what nutrients are in short supply. Here is a chart that may be helpful.

< 162 >

Nutrient deficiency	Common symptoms
Vitamin B12	Short-term memory loss, sore tongue, fatigue, burning/tingling feet
Magnesium	Muscle spasm, chronic migraines, recurrent eyelid twitch, heart flutter, back aches, anxiety reactions, leg cramps, constipation, monthly cramping in females
Zinc	Altered taste, poor appetite, poor immunity, poor night vision
Iron	Fatigue, cold hands and feet, pale skin, sleep apnea, crave acid foods (tomatoes) and ice chips
Vitamin C	Easy skin bruising, bleeding gums, fatigue, anemia
Coenzyme Q10	Chronic cough
Vitamin A	Diminished night vision
Folic acid	Abnormal pap smear, mental depression, memory problems

Question: Should I always buy chelated minerals?

Answer: Consumers ask about chelated minerals under the false assumption that greater absorption is better. The body does a good job of limiting the absorption of minerals since over-mineralization can be troublesome in both the short and long term. For example, if the body absorbed all the calcium from high-dose supplements it would over-alkalize the blood circulation. The body has a mechanism that halts absorption beyond 500 mg of calcium consumed at a time to prevent this from occurring. Only a small amount of iron, copper and zinc are actually absorbed. In the long term, excessive copper and iron may result in overload, particularly in males and postmenopausal females.

Mineral overload can occur in a relatively short period of time, just a few weeks. For example, males who consume iron-rich red meat with alcoholic beverages, which increases iron absorption, are at greater risk for iron overload and liver problems. Minerals are also in a dynamic balance.

< 163 >

Minerals compete for absorption, such as calcium and magnesium and zinc and copper, so balanced mineral formulas are strongly suggested. For example, for every 10 milligrams of supplemental zinc an additional milligram of copper is needed to prevent a rise in cholesterol. Supplemental mineral absorption is also enhanced by taking them with meals.

On the other hand, no sense purchasing poorly absorbed minerals, like the mineral oxides which are generally considered the poorest-absorbed form of minerals. For example, mineral sulfates are better absorbed than oxides. Mineral gluconates are also superior to oxides. Calcium citrate requires no stomach acid for absorption and exhibits superior absorption qualities over calcium carbonate. Recognize that minerals are positively charged ions and attach to negatively-charged ions as their carriers. The total amount in a mineral complex may be 400 milligrams, of which only 120 milligrams is elemental mineral and the rest is its carrier.

Accelerated aging could be defined as the accumulation of excess minerals. During the growth years minerals have a place to go, calcium to the bones and iron to bone marrow to produce new red blood cells. But once full growth is achieved, then the body doesn't quite need as much calcium and iron. However, females may become pregnant and then they would donate their iron and calcium to their developing offspring which prevents overload. When not pregnant, menstruating females will control their iron through their monthly cycle since blood loss causes a loss of circulating iron. Once women reach menopause or undergo an early hysterectomy they lose this protection and accumulate iron like adult males. A 40-year old male will have twice the stored iron levels as a 40-year old female and will also have twice the rate of diabetes, cancer, heart disease and infections. Women universally outlive males due to their ability to control iron stores.

< 164 >

The 17 essential minerals:
Calcium
Phosphorus
Potassium
Sodium
Chloride
Magnesium
Magnesium
Sulfur
Boron
Chromium
Copper
Iodine
Manganese
Molybdenem
Selenium
Silicon
Zinc

Question: What about coral calcium? Is it a superior form of calcium?

Answer: Coral calcium sourced from Okinawa has recently been widely promoted. Its claim of superior absorption does not stand up to scrutiny. The percentage of coral calcium available for absorption is published in advertisements at 39 percent, and for coral mineral powder at 84 to 98 percent. However the body maintains a tight control over the absorption of calcium. More than 500 milligrams of calcium in a single serving is poorly absorbed. Too much calcium and the blood circulation would become too alkaline. If 80 to 90 percent of calcium were absorbed, there would be undesirable health consequences, including an electrolyte imbalance which could induce a spasm in heart muscle leading to sudden-death heart attack.

Another misleading claim is made that calcium alkalizes the body. Actually every form of calcium is alkaline and shifts the body away

< 165 >

from an acid state. Coral calcium is not unique in that respect; ditto for magnesium.

Coral calcium is calcium carbonate. It is an array of 73 minerals, not just calcium, and contains heavy metals. Most coral calcium products do not reveal they more than double the amount of aluminum intake from the diet. Aluminum appears to interfere with the absorption of calcium. [Ann Endocrinology 50: 40-43, 1989] Aluminum is a powerful nerve toxin. [Brain Research Bulletin 55: 187-96, 2001] Generally, aluminum in the diet and in coral calcium is very poorly absorbed. Aluminum absorption from drinking water is very low (0.3%). [Toxicology 161: 93-101, 2001] People on Okinawa obtain their coral calcium largely from drinking water, not supplements. But when aluminum is combined with fluoridated tap water it can become soluble and increase the amount of potentially toxic aluminum in brain tissues. [Behavioral Neuroal Biology 61: 233-41, 1994; Brain Research 784: 284-98, 1998; Food Additive Contamination 18: 515-23, 2001] Both fluoride and citrate (as in calcium citrate) increase the absorption of aluminum and lead from dietary sources. [Bone Mineralization 20: 87-97, 1993; Research Communication Molecular Pathology Pharmacology 91: 225-31, 1996] Some calcium carbonate supplements have also been found to contain lead, another potential nerve toxin. [Environmental Health Perspectives 109: 283-88, 2001] However, calcium citrate without aluminum does not pose a risk of toxicity to people with normal functioning kidneys. [Bone Mineralization 20: 87-97, 1993] Bone mineral formulas should be free of heavy metals so there is no potential long-term toxicity.

An unfounded claim is made for coral calcium as a longevity factor. It is assumed that the longevity on Okinawa is solely due to coral calcium intake. In fact, it is the slow accumulation of calcium that is a marker of accelerated aging after full bone growth and mineralization is achieved after about age 18. Calcium accumulates in blood vessels, the kidneys (stones), the eyes and heart valves with advancing age.

The promoters of coral calcium claim there is no problem with getting too much calcium. They cite the Masai tribe in Africa that consumes

< 166 >

about 6000 milligrams per day, mostly from milk, as evidence of the safety of calcium. However, the Masai only live to about 40 years of age, not nearly the longevity of people on the island of Okinawa where coral calcium originates. It is obvious that the diet of the Masai, which also plentiful in whole grains which contain a natural mineral chelator (IP6 phytic acid) and their widespread lactose intolerance (62% of Masai tribes people), limits their calcium absorption and spares them from the problems of calcium overload. [American Journal Clinical Nutrition, 32:779-82, 1979]

Another widespread myth is that coral calcium protects against diabetes. Actually, diabetes has been defined as a disease of excessive calcium influx into cells. There is a relative high rate of diabetes among the people of Okinawa who are purported to consume large amounts of coral calcium in drinking water. [Hypertension Research 2002 25: 185-90, 2002]

It is interesting that the book THE OKINAWA FACTOR (2001), written by Drs. Bradley and Craig Wilcox and Dr. Makoto Suzuki, notes that women on Okinawa who live to be 100 years of age only consume about 400 to 625 milligrams of calcium per day (page 144).

Question: Should consumers look for the USP approval seal on vitamins?

Answer: The United States Pharmacopeia (USP) established guidelines for the dissolution of vitamin and mineral tablets. Unlike gelatin capsules, tablets are compressed into small hard bricks using binding agents. Tablets may or may not dissolve in the digestive tract, particularly among old adults who do not produce enough stomach acid. If the tablets don't break down, nutrients will not be adequately absorbed and the pill will pass through the digestive tract intact. The USP standards for dissolution do not apply to gelatin capsules, only tablets. Pharmaceutical standards means tablets must dissolve within 15 to 30 minutes in the digestive tract. A crude test is to place clear vinegar in a dish and drop in a vitamin or mineral pill. It should break down and dissolve within 15 to 30 minutes to meet USP standards.

< 167 >

At the current time the USP is attempting to set standards to ensure the labelled amount of an active ingredient is provided in vitamin and mineral pills. Soon some brands of single vitamins and minerals may display the USP logo which guarantees the product contains what the label claims. However, this will obviously increase costs to consumers to comply with testing. The ability to economically test every ingredient in multivitamin and mineral supplements that may contain 30 or more nutrients may be cost prohibitive.

Question: What about the claim that calcium, in particular coral calcium, alkalizes the body's tissues and helps prevent cancer?
Answer: This theory started with Otto Warberg, a German biochemist. [Science 123: 309-14, 1956] Warberg was the first to find that there is abnormal metabolism in cancer cells and they produce acidity, for which Warberg was awarded two Nobel prizes. Recently researchers have found that tumor cells are actually very alkaline, not acid. [Novartis Found Symposium 240: 46-62, 2001; J Theoretical Biol 196: 237-50, 1999] However, the area surrounding a tumor is acid. Tumor cells lack cell energy and cannot adequately pump out sodium and calcium from their insides. Therefore, tumor cells are overloaded with calcium, which is alkaline, not the other way around. Lacking energy, cancer cells switch from utilizing oxygen to fermentation of sugar to produce energy. This process produces lactic acid which is expelled from the cell. Therefore, the area surrounding cancer cells is acidic, not the cancer cell itself. Any effort to alkalize the area outside the tumor cell would be useless since the tumor cells continue to expel acid. The best approach may be to supplement with coenzyme Q10 which helps to restore cellular energy and has been shown in some studies to causes tumors to go into complete remission. [Biochem Biophys Res Comm 199: 1504-08, 1994; 212: 172-77, 1995; Molecular Aspects Med 15: 231-40S, 1994]

Question: Does vitamin E, as alpha tocopherol, lower cholesterol?
Answer: Alpha tocopherol, the common form of vitamin E in vitamin pills, slightly elevates the coenzyme A enzyme in the liver that produces cholesterol. So, no, vitamin E does not reduce cholesterol. Tocotrienols,

< 168 >

another vitamin E-like molecule, have an opposite effect. [Atherosclerosis 161: 199-207, 2002]

In an animal study, a tocotrienol mixture reduced atherosclerotic plaques two times better than alpha tocopherol. [J Nutrition 131: 2606-18, 2001] Tocotrienols are better antioxidants, by 40 to 60 times, than tocopherols, though they don't replace the essential need for tocopherols. [Journal Nutrition 131: 369S, 2001]

Tocotrienols, like statin drugs, reduce cholesterol by inhibiting an enzyme called coenzyme A reductase. [Journal Nutrition 131: 369S, 2001] However, unlike statin drugs, tocotrienols help raise coenzyme Q10 levels.

Because tocotrienols are believed to convert into tocopherols in high doses, the provision of excessive amounts of tocotrienols may be counter productive. In humans, a 100 milligram dose of tocotrienols appears to be the maximum dose to decrease cholesterol (-20%), LDL cholesterol (-25%), and triglycerides (-12%). [Atherosclerosis 161: 199-207, 2002]

Question: What can't some people tolerate vitamin pills?
Answer: Many people have "leaky gut syndrome." They take vitamin pills, they don't agree with them, they experience uncomfortable symptoms and they abandon use of vitamins. The problem is not the vitamin pills but the state of health of the digestive tract. Leaky gut is involved in colitis and Crohn's disease. Chronic inflammation and irritation break down the protective mucus coating of the digestive tract and widens the gaps in between cells. This permits undigested proteins to enter the circulatory system which then triggers the immune system. Pain, diarrhea, vomiting, rashes, may develop. The most common causes of "leaky gut" are alcohol or anti-inflammatory drugs like aspirin, ibuprofen or acetaminophen. [Gut 49: 650-55, 2001] Tobacco actually tightens the junctions in the mucus lining of the digestive tract, so people who stop smoking may actually notice problems with "leaky gut." It has been observed that the spouses of people with Crohn's disease have more leaky gut problems than spouses of healthy individuals. [Am J Gastroent

< 169 >

96: 2934-38, 2001] So obviously some common irritant is involved. Natural anti-inflammatory agents such as quercetin, ginger, green tea, may be helpful in these conditions. Also, high dose zinc, glutathione and good bacteria (acidophilus) may be helpful in calming down an irritated gut. [Am J Gastroent 97: 2000-04, 2002; Dig Dis Sci 47: 511-16, 2002; Inflamm Bowel Dis 7: 94-98, 2001; Pharm Res 19: 602-08, 2002]

Question: I take a multivitamin, but I still feel fatigued. What should I do?

Answer: Here is a quick guide to nutritional approaches to fatigue:

1. Pernicious anemia, usually poor absorption of vitamin B12; usually accompanied by fatigue, short-term memory loss, sore tongue, burning, tingling feet; take up to 3000 mcg of vitamin B12 preferably as methylcobalamin.

2. Low thyroid, usually accompanied by weight gain. Underarm temperature below 98 degrees F upon waking in AM is usually sign of low metabolism; thyroid may need iron, omega-3 oils, iodine, selenium. Gugulipid is an herb which may boost thyroid function.

3. Iron-deficiency anemia, usually accompanied by pale skin, cold hands and feet, craving for acidic foods (tomatoes), poor concentration, need to take naps. Eat red meat or supplement the daily diet for six weeks with Ferronyl (carbonyl) iron then only once weekly (if at all) thereafter).

4. Weak heart, usually accompanied by ankle swelling. Supplement with coenzyme Q10 100-300 mg.

5. Poor adrenal function, usually accompanied by weak immune system and chronic illnesses and infections; supplement with vitamin B5 pantothenic acid 25-100 mg (royal jelly also provides good natural source of vitamin B5); vitamin C 500-2000 mg; flaxseed oil or omega-3 fish oil 2000-3000 mg.

6. Iron overload, usually accompanied by frequent infections, skin discoloration, elevated liver enzymes and elevated cholesterol, high blood sugar; more common among males or females who have undergone early hysterectomy. Chelate (remove) excess iron by using IP6 rice bran extract for 30-600 days with water only on empty stomach, 1600-2400 mg.

< 170 >

Where to Find Multivitamins that Meet These Requirements?

You are going to have a difficult time finding multivitamins that meet all of these requirements. Only now are vitamin manufacturers beginning to respond to changes in nutritional science. Use the following checklist as your purchasing guide.

Is your multivitamin complete? Potent? Balanced?

Checklist for Multivitamins 25 Things To Look For In Multivitamins Rate Your Own Multi
POTENCY
500 mg vitamin C
No more than 200-300 IU vitamin E
6 mg lutein/zeaxanthin
800 mcg folic acid
800 IU vitamin D3
300 mcg vitamin B12
BALANCE
Calcium and magnesium- near equal or more mag over cal
Zinc and copper 10-to-1 ratio zinc over copper
Alpha, beta, delta and gamma forms of tocopherols and tocotrienols
Carotenoids: beta carotene, lutein/zeaxanthin, near equal ratios
Bioflavonoids equalling 70% of vitamin C
FORMS OF NUTRIENTS
SelenoExcel organic selenium
Natural d-alpha tocopherol vitamin E rather than synthetic dl-alpha tocopherol
Vitamin B12 as methylcobalamin

< 171 >

	Calcium as citrate
	Vitamin C as mineral ascorbates
	INCLUSION
	Sulfur (taurine, lipoic acid, glutathione)
	Boron 3 mg or more
	Chromium 200 mcg
	Coenzyme Q10
	RESTRICTIONS
	No iron, copper
	No more than 10 mg riboflavin (vitamin B2)
	Beta carotene rather than formed vitamin A
	DELIVERY AND ABSORPTION
	Inclusion of enzymes
	Easy-to-absorb capsules rather than tablets

Rating the multivitamins

People who take multivitamins on a regular basis certainly know they are the <u>best bargain for the informed supplement buyer</u>. The separate purchase of each nutrient in a multivitamin would be too costly for most consumers. Multivitamins eliminate the need to take so many pills in a day.

<u>Where supplement manufacturers have disappointed is their inability to respond to new developments in the science of vitamins and minerals</u>. Most companies take the role of follower, buying into false arguments over potential overdosage and Tolerable Upper Limits (which are actually entirely safe upper limits), or copying what other companies have done. Consumers want results from the vitamin and mineral products they use. They may not experience the many benefits they hear about in the news media simply because they are taking the wrong multivitamin. <u>Consumers have a strong chance of selecting an inferior brand of multivitamin simply because the majority of brands offered are poorly formulated</u>. Of the 49 brands included in this multivitamin survey, only

< 172 >

8 brands scored better than 40 points out of 100 and only one brand scored better than 50 points.

While Americans think of vitamins as promoting health, they may fail to recognize that poorly-made vitamin and mineral preparations may be causing the very health problems they experience. Liver disease from iron overload, sudden-death heart attack, cataracts, high cholesterol are just some of the consequences of taking poorly formulated multivitamins.

The learning curve on vitamins isn't easy and usually the health benefits of vitamins and minerals are learned one at a time. Timid supplement users may be reticent about getting into multivitamins for budgetary reasons or unsurety about over-dosing with mega vitamins or potential conflicts with medications. If this book has taught readers anything it should be that concerns involving overdosage are mostly fabricated or poorly founded. The most costly multivitamin consumers can buy is a poorly formulated one that doesn't deliver on its health promises.

This third survey of major brands of multivitamins has been discouraging if for no other reason than the remarkable breakthroughs in nutritional science have largely been ignored by multivitamin manufacturers. In just the past three years or so it has become apparent that human health would be enhanced if more folic acid (800 mcg from supplements) could be consumed. It is apparent that larger doses of vitamin D (800 mcg from supplements) effectively reduce the risk of bone fractures among older Americans and reduce the need for more and more supplemental calcium which is problematic. A giant u-turn has taken place regarding vitamin E as researchers have identified the need for the full family of vitamin E molecules (tocopherols and tocotrienols) and an optimal dose for alpha tocopherol (around 200 IU), less than many consumers now consume. These are remarkable developments. They should be incorporated into well-made multivitamins.

Twenty-five different factors were surveyed in multivitamins regarding dosage, type of nutrients, such as calcium citrate which is preferred over calcium carbonate and the full array of amino acid-bound selenium

< 173 >

molecules (SelenoExcel™) is preferred over inorganic selenate or selenite. Some multivitamin brands are missing key ingredients, such as lutein and tocotrienols. Some manufacturers frankly appear to be oblivious to the potential hazards posed by excessive iron, riboflavin and the fatty form of vitamin A.

The twenty-five desirable factors in multivitamins were compared against what various products actually say they deliver on their labels. Each factor was worth 4 points. A perfect score would be 100. The majority of the $10 a month multivitamins, which scored 12 points or less out of 100, are being sold in drug stores. A pharmacist couldn't even make a good recommendation to most consumers for multivitamins simply because there are only poorly-rated brands on their shelves. These are the very multivitamins that the American Medical Association mistakenly says are sufficient to meet the nutritional needs of the American population that largely doesn't consume the recommended five servings of daily fruits and vegetables. This book reveals that these poorly-formulated but economical multivitamins, when combined with typical dietary intake, do not even provide the amount of nutrients found in a plant-food based diet, the gold standard for comparison.

At the other end of the scale, multivitamins selling for *"Cadillac"* prices often don't offer much more than other mid-priced brands. One product, offered by a well known nutritionist, requires 10 pills be taken per day at a monthly retail price exceeding $100! For less than a dollar a day consumer can purchase the best rated multivitamin, which may be the best health insurance one can buy.

Here are the results of the latest survey:

< 174 >

RANK 2003 Survey	MULTIVITAMIN 53 Brands	MANUFACTURER	# PILLS PER DAY	SCORE (100 IS BEST)
1	Purity Perfect Multi	Purity Products	4 capsules	88
2	Synergy Ultra	Nutraceutical Sciences Institute	22 capsules	68
3	Elan Vital	Source Naturals	6 tablets	44
3	Health Pack	USANA	Daily pack	44
3	Gary Null's Supreme Health	Gary Null	10 tablets	44
4	Maxilife Co Q10 Formula	Twinlab	4 capsules	40
4	Life Extension Mix	Life Extension	14 capsules	40
4	Cooper Complete	Cooper Wellness	4 tablets	40
5	Pathway Basic Nutrition	Abundant Nutrition	4 capsules	40
5	Essentials	USANA	6 tablets	36
5	Stop Aging Now	Jean Carper	6 tablets	36
5	Mega Antioxidant	USANA	3 tablets	36
6	Life Force Multiple	Source Naturals	2 capsules	32
6	Just Once Multivitamin	Rainbow Light	1 tablet	32
7	Daily Advantage	Dr. Williams	4 capsules	28
7	Ultra-High Absorb	Swanson	1 capsule	28
7	Advanced Nutrition System	Rainbow Light	6 tablets	28
7	Omnium	Solgar	2 tablets	28
7	Ocudyne II	Nutricology	2 capsules	28
8	Prime Years	Schiff	1 softgel	24
8	Forward Plus	Dr. Whitaker	Daily pack	24
8	Super One Daily	Carlson Labs	1 tablet	24
8	Nutrilite	Access Business Group	1 tablet	24
8	Multi 1-to-3	Jarrow Formulas	3 tablets	24
9	Daily Multi	Swanson	1 capsule	20
9	Super Multi	Linus Pauling	3 caplets	20
9	Essential Life Daily	Country Life	3 tablets	20
9	Multivitamin	Nature's Way	3 capsules	20

< 175 >

RANK 2003 Survey	MULTIVITAMIN 53 Brands	MANUFACTURER	# PILLS PER DAY	SCORE (100 IS BEST)
9	Special Two	Now Foods	2 tablets	20
10	Mega Vita Gel	Puritan's Pride	2 softgels	16
10	My Favorite Multiple	Natrol	4 tablets	16
10	Superior One Plus	Swanson	1 tablet	16
10	Vit-Min +75	Now Foods	1 tablet	16
10	Century Formula	Swanson	1 tablet	16
11	One-A-Day Men's	One-A-Day	1 tablet	12
11	No Iron Multi	Nature's Way	3 capsules	12
11	High Potency Ultra Vita Man	Vitamin World	1 tablet	12
11	Vita Lea	Shaklee Corp	2 tablets	12
11	Daily One Caps	Twinlab	1 capsule	12
11	Centrum Silver	Lederle	1 tablet	12
11	Ultra Mega Gold	GNC	2 tablets	12
11	Kirkland Daily Multivitamin	Costco	1 tablet	12
12	Central Vite	Rite Aid	1 tablet	8
12	Essential Daily	Nature Made	1 tablet	8
12	Whole Source	Rite-Aid	1 tablet	8
12	Multivitamins	Vitamin Shoppe	Packet	8
12	Premium	Kirkland	1 tablet	8
12	Geritol Complete	GlaxoSmithKline	1 tablet	8
12	Mega Min	Puritan's Pride	1 tablet	8
12	Theragran M Advanced	Mead Johnson	1 caplet	8
12	ABC Plus Senior	Nature's Bounty	1 tablet	8
13	Ultra Vita-Min	Puritan's Pride	1 tablet	4
13	Centrum Select	Lederle	1 tablet	4
13	CVS Mega Multi	CVS	1 tablet	4

Bill Sardi's Ranking of Multivitamins 2003 survey Copyright Bill Sardi 2003

< 176 >

Recommended suppliers of multivitamins

Purity Products
139 Haven Avenue
Port Washington, New York 11050
Purchase online at a discount at www.purityproducts.com
Toll free: 888-313 7873

Source Naturals
Source Naturals doesn't sell directly to consumers.
Consumers may purchase products from one of our many retailers, or purchase online.
Customer Service: 831-438-1144
Toll-free: 800-815-2333
Address: 19 Janis Way
Scotts Valley, CA 95066
Fax: 831-438-7410
International Sales Information:
Located at Threshold Enterprises, Ltd.
Headquarters in Scotts Valley, CA
E-mail: thresholdent@hotmail.com
Telephone: 831-461-7325
Fax: 831-461-9573

Twin Laboratories Inc.
150 Motor Parkway
Suite 210
Hauppauge, NY 11788
Phone: 631-467-3140
Product Information
at Twin Laboratories Inc.
Product inquiries
Catalogs / Literature requests
Special requests or inquiries
product@twinlab.com
Fax: 631-467-2973

< 177 >

Addendum
What Is the Antioxidant Power of Your Diet and Supplements?

Americans hear a lot about antioxidants these days. How much antioxidant power do your foods plus dietary supplements provide?

Before this question is answered it would be helpful to gain an understanding of your need for antioxidant protection, which varies from individual to individual.

What generates "rusting" free radicals in the body?

First, we need to understand what generates oxidation in the body. The oxygen you breathe, the fat and iron/copper content of your meals, the frequency and calorie content of meals, and your age, to a large extent determine the amount of *"rusting"* going on in your body. Exercise, infection and exposure to radiation (solar, x-rays) also increase oxidation.

Oxygen is a necessary and good thing in the human body, but also a potentially harmful factor. While much is made of toxins in the air, ranging from smog to radon gas, it is **oxygen itself that is the primary toxin in the body.** About 4 percent of the oxygen humans breathe converts into a toxic byproduct called an oxygen free radical. These oxygen radicals are the *"rusting agents"* of the body. Exposure to greater than 21% oxygen can produce injurious side effects. Pure O_2 for as little as six hours can cause chest soreness, cough and sore throat. High oxygen levels in incubators produces blindness in babies. [Nutrition Reviews 52: 253-65, 1994] The faddish *"oxygen bars"* that once received publicity, where people would come into a bar for a drink while inhaling oxygen through a nasal tube, improves oxygenation of tissues but also can be problematic. That is why antioxidants (anti-rusting agents) are

< 178 >

widely promoted in plant foods and dietary supplements to counter aging, improve immunity from disease and to promote health.

While oxygen (O_2) and naturally-produced hydrogen peroxide (H_2O_2) are sources of rusting in the human body, they are not very reactive until they are brought into contact with **unbound metals**

> **A 1993 issue of the Journal of the American Medical Association conceded that "all human disease has some relationship with free radical species."**
> [J Am Med Assoc 270: 2024, 1993]

such as iron and copper which then generate the most powerful of all rusting agents, the dreaded **hydroxyl radical** which attacks and damages almost everything found in the human body. [Nutrition Reviews 55: 44-52S, 1997] The hydroxyl radical is believed to be the toxicant that triggers genetic mutations that leads to cancer.

Since DNA damage is considered the initial event in cancer, **the importance of DNA protection from oxidative damage becomes paramount.** Supplementation with 100 mg of vitamin C, 100 mg (~100 IU) of vitamin E, 6 mg of beta carotene and 50 mcg of selenium has been shown to reduce breaks in chromosomes by half with an even greater effect in smokers. [Mutagenesis 18: 371-76, 2003]

Researchers at the University of California at Berkeley estimate that **the number of oxidative hits to DNA per cell per day is about 10,000 in humans.** Enzymes can repair most but not all the breaks in strands of DNA in human cells. DNA damage accumulates with advancing age. There is a greater need for antioxidants with advancing age. The *"flame"* of oxidation in the body increases with advancing age and is associated with unsuccessful aging (disability, disease). [J Am Geriatrics Society 44: 823-27, 1996] In **old age there are about 2 million DNA breaks per cell per day!** [Proceedings Nat'l Academy Sciences 90: 7915-22, 1993] Think of this as bullets riddling your cells with destruction. The cells can rebuild, but the repair process may not be able to keep up.

< 179 >

MEASURE OF OXIDIZED
LIVER DNA

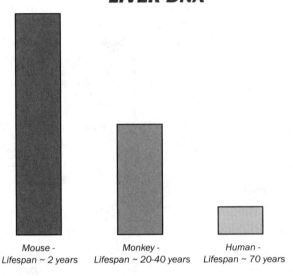

| Mouse -
Lifespan ~ 2 years | Monkey -
Lifespan ~ 20-40 years | Human -
Lifespan ~ 70 years |

Oxidative by-products in liver DNA may determine lifespan of mammals.

One intriguing study shows that the lifespan of various mammals is dependent upon a marker of oxidation in liver DNA. Mice, which only live about 2 years, exhibit high levels of oxidative by-products in their livers, whereas monkeys which live 20-40 years have half as much toxic byproducts and humans who live about 70 years about 1/8th as much. [Am J Clin Nut 53: 373-79S, 1991] So limitation of oxidation may help control longevity, or it just may be a marker and not an age controlling agent at all. There is still a lot to learn. In one study vitamin E and strawberry supplements reduced oxidative byproducts in the livers of mice but did not affect maximum life span. [Annals NY Academy Sci 20: 854-60, 1998] So gaining an understanding of these dynamic factors can be perplexing.

Reducing the need for antioxidants by limiting food

Calorie restricted diets, or fasting, reduce the *"flame"* of oxidation in living tissues. Another way of saying this is, **the less food you eat the less antioxidants you need from foods and supplements to counter adverse effects of free radicals.** [Arch Biochem Biophysics 333: 189-97,

< 180 >

1996] This obviously validates the idea of fasting. Even brief fasts are beneficial.

Food stokes the fires of free radical production and Americans generally eat a lot of food, about 3700+ calories per day. (For comparison, the long-lived Japanese consume about 2800 calories and the Japanese on Okinawa consume only about 1100-1500 calories per day. Okinawa is where many are living beyond the age of 100 years in good health.) With about 40% of the US population consuming fat-laden fast foods on a daily basis, there is a great need to counter the adverse effects posed by over-consumption with antioxidants. [J Am Dietetic Assn 103: 1332-38, 2003]

The best advice is to **take antioxidant supplements with meals, when the "flame" of oxidation is high.** The provision of high dose vitamins C and E has been shown to counter the adverse effects after consumption of a sugar or fat-laden meal. [University at Buffalo, American Diabetes Association, June 16, 2002]

A high-fat meal impairs the ability of blood vessels to widen (control blood pressure) for at least 4 hours after a meal. The provision of a powdered fruit-vegetable concentrate can reverse this effect. [J Am College Cardiology 41: 1744-49, 2003]

This is in contrast to another study which showed that 1000 mg of vitamin C and 800 IU of vitamin E did <u>not</u> improve blood flow following consumption of a high or low-fat meal. [Journal Am Med Assn 278: 1682-86, 1997]

Why didn't the high-dose antioxidant vitamins work while the plant-food concentrate was effective?

Here is an important point. According to the US Department of Agriculture, **the iron and copper binding molecules called polyphenols in fruits (in particular grapes, berries, cherries, olives, cocoa, tea and citrus rind) account for most of the antioxidant capacity of fruits and**

< 181 >

vegetables. [J AOAC Int 83: 950-56, 2000] A plentiful supply of polyphenols may or may not be provided in the best plant food diet or supplement regimen. Interestingly, a major measure of oxidation is not reduced among vegetarians compared to nonvegetarians. [European J Epidemiology 11: 207-11, 1995] Even dedicated herbivores may not get enough antioxidants.

Even most multivitamins do not provide a significant amount of polyphenols (sometimes called bioflavonoids) either. Maybe, even with mega doses of vitamins C and E, multivitamins just don't have enough antioxidant punch. In comparative studies, vitamin E did not affect markers of DNA damage in liver cells, but green tea, which contains polyphenols, did. [Free Radical Research 25: 57-74, 1996]

Certainly Americans are likely to consume antioxidant-poor plant foods. The most popular plant foods consumed by Americans (in order of consumption) are iceberg lettuce, tomatoes, French fries, orange juice and onions.

So how many servings of antioxidant-rich plant foods do we need to consume per day? When 25 men consumed 5-7 servings of fruits and vegetables or an equivalent in plant food concentrates their antioxidant blood levels rose but a chemical marker of oxidation was not affected. [British J Nutrition 85: 459-64, 2001] Does this mean humans need far more antioxidants than most optimal diets and supplement regimens provide?

The mixed message

So now that you are all set to load up on antioxidants, especially the polyphenols, here is the current mistaken advice you are reading in the lay press. A Los Angeles Times article published late last year said: *"In recent years, several larger research studies have found that people who took antioxidant supplements received no greater protection from chronic diseases than those who didn't... They are no longer considered the miracle cure they once were."* [LA Times Oct 27, 2003] The LA Times article cited a study

< 182 >

of more than 20,000 British adults who took antioxidant supplements but showed no difference in heart attack, stroke or cancer rates compared to people who took a worthless placebo tablet. So the LA Times concluded by saying *"For now, many doctors and scientists agree that you're better off consuming antioxidants in their natural form --- by eating fruits and vegetables --- than by taking a vitamin pill."* Melanie Polk, director of nutrition education at the American Institute of Cancer Research ended by saying: *"We should be spending our money in the produce department, not the vitamin aisle."* There is always an element of truth in these news reports. Could it be that antioxidant supplements, in particular multivitamins, simply don't provide enough antioxidant power? Are the vitamin supplement nay-sayers correct?

> **Even small incremental increases in fruit and vegetable consumption yields potential health benefits. Just an increase of 1.4 servings of plant foods has been shown to lower systolic blood pressure (the first pressure number) by 4 points, equal to what some drugs accomplish.**
> [Lancet 359: 1969-74, 2002]

Run to the vegetable stand?

OK, OK, we're all headed to the vegetable stand. The impetus to increase fruit and vegetable consumption arose over a decade ago when a review of over 200 scientific studies revealed plant food consumption decreases the risk of cancer. Additionally, every serving of plant food reduces a person's risk for heart disease by 4 percent. So the American Cancer Institute developed its 5-a-day program. [J Am Dietetic Assn 94: 32-36, 1994] However, human compliance has been low. A study of 15,000 US adults revealed only 17% consumed 5 or more servings of fruits and vegetables. [J Am Dietetic Assn 99: 1241-48, 1999]

< 183 >

But horrors, **the 5-a-day program has met failure also.** We know that low dietary intake of fruits and vegetables doubles the risk for most types of cancer. [Proceedings Nat'l Academy Sciences 90: 7915-22, 1993] But high consumption of plant foods doesn't necessarily lower the risk of cancer either. Maybe now we understand why. It could be lack of those important phytonutrients, from dark-green vegetables and in particular the polyphenols in fruits.

It's now a decade later and the National Cancer Institute (NCI) can't report its 5-a-day program has dented the rate of cancer. So it has launched its updated version of its plant food campaign --- 9-a-day. **Five servings is "just the bare minimum,"** says the NCI. **Only 4 percent of US males consume 9 servings a day!** [British Medical Journal 326: 1003, 2003] While the vegetables provide important antioxidants like the folic acid (required for DNA repair), lutein, beta carotene and lycopene, it is the fruits that provide the all important iron-binding antioxidants, the polyphenols. [J Nutrition 130: 3063-67, 2000]

High antioxidant foods

To help sort out which foods have the most antioxidant power, the US Department of Agriculture developed a measure of the combined antioxidant power of foods and supplements. It's called the Oxygen Radical Absorption Capacity (ORAC). Throw all the plant foods you eat into a pile and how much *"anti-rusting"* power do you get? The consumption of 5 servings of plant foods yields about 1750 ORAC units, and 9-servings about 3150 ORAC units. Here is a comparison of the ORAC values of various plant foods.

< 184 >

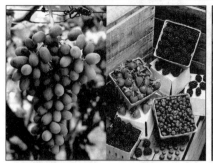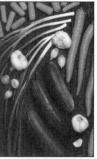

High ORAC antioxidant plant foods   Lower ORAC
(provide iron-binding polyphenols)   antioxidant
                                                     vegetables

Plant food	ORAC antioxidant values per milligram	Increase in ORAC antioxidant power over broccoli, carrots or barley
Broccoli, carrots, barley	Reference for comparison	---
Garlic, nettles, onion	0.05	1.25 times
Spinach, kale	0.07	1.70 times
Melon seed	0.10	2.50 times
Cherry	0.29	7.25 times
Red wine grape	0.30	7.50 times
Blueberry	0.40	10.00 times
Pomegranate	0.45	11.25 times
Grape seed	8.00	200.00 times
Apple peel	15.0	375.00 times

Most health conscious Americans simply are not going to be able to consume nine servings of fruits and veges a day, certainly not on a consistent basis. Is there any shortcut? Yes, we can juice. But people who juice often use vegetable green drinks rather than the polyphenol-rich fruits. Certainly, fresh food should not be shunned for a pill or a greens drink. But there is a crying need for more ORAC anti-oxidant power in multivitamins to make up for any shortages in the diet.

< 185 >

Multivitamin antioxidant power

Just how much ORAC antioxidant power do multivitamins provide? Various brands of multivitamins were selected based upon their labels which advertised extra antioxidant potency or inclusion of plant extracts. They were tested for ORAC antioxidant power by Genox, an independent laboratory. The results are shown on the chart to the right.

This chart shows that the addition of antioxidant-rich fruit (polyphenol) extracts to a multivitamin, compacted into just one extra capsule per day, can make a big difference in delivery of antioxidant power, equivalent in this case to 15.5 servings of fruits and vegetables (5450 ORAC units).

Bottom line: Eat the high ORAC antioxidant-rich fruits (apple peel, grapes, pomegranates, cherries, blueberries. Juicing may be advantageous but poses challenges in having to consume high volumes of food and maintaining fresh stocks in the kitchen. Greens formulas (drinks, powders) may or may not be advantageous and should be labeled for their ORAC values to help consumers evaluate their antioxidant power. The addition of a relatively small amount of fruit extracts to a 5-capsule a day multivitamin regimen could deliver the ORAC antioxidant power needed when the body is challenged by oxidative stress.

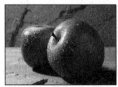 Apples provide about 8-12 milligrams of vitamin C which represents less than one percent of the total antioxidants in apples. Most of the antioxidant power of an apple is found in the peel. [Am J Clin Nutrition 78: 517-20S, 2003]

< 186 >

BRAND OF MULTIVITAMIN	ANTIOXIDANT ORAC UNITS
Health food store brand-NP	88.5
Supermarket brand- C	92.2
Health food store brand - NL	123.1
Health food store brand -T	137.0
Health food store brand-SN	151.2
Health food store brand- N	151.9
Health Food Store Brand- MF	188.1
Health Food Store brand- NL2	197.5
Health Food Store brand -NW	291.3
Purity Perfect Multivitamin – Purity Products (4 caps/day)	342.4
ORAC antioxidant score – 5 servings fruits & veges	1750.0
ORAC antioxidant score – 9 servings fruits & veges	3150.0
Purity Perfect Multi Super Greens Formula (5 caps/day)	5450.0

Tests conducted by independent laboratories: Genox and Brunswick

The above chart ranks some brands of multivitamins by their total ORAC antioxidant power. Most brands don't even provide the ORAC value of one serving of plant foods. The addition of selected antioxidant-rich plant extracts can make a dramatic difference in total antioxidant power. An example is Purity Products Perfect Multivitamin which provides some plant extracts and herbs (ORAC score 342.4) compared to the same product with added fruit-based polyphenols and green vegetable extracts (Purity Products Perfect Multi Super Greens Formula) which exhibits an incredible ORAC score of 5450.0, equivalent to 15.5 servings of fruits and vegetables). Chart as of 5/04.

< 187 >

Index

< 188 >

< 189 >

< 190 >

< 191 >

< 192 >

< 193 >

NOTES

< 194 >

NOTES

< 195 >

Other Publications by Bill Sardi

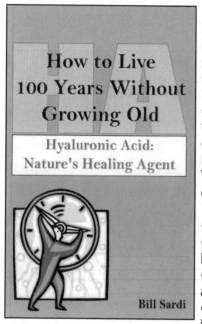

How to Live 100 Years Without Growing Old

Hyaluronic Acid: Nature's Healing Agent

Bill Sardi

Hyaluronic acid is a revolutionary natural molecule that stops or even reverses aging. Spanish explorer Juan Ponce de Leon (early 1500s) searched for the "fountain of youth," crystal waters that natives claimed would instantly endow immortal youth and beauty. Hyaluronic acid is the modern day "fountain of youth." What does it do?

• HA holds water in the body.
• HA acts as a lubricant in the heart valves.
• HA is the spongy shock absorber at the ends of bones.
• HA holds most of the moisture in the skin.
• HA makes up 80 percent of the human eye.
• HA provides a barrier against the spread of infection.
• HA helps to erase fine facial aging lines and wrinkles (plastic surgery in a bottle).
• HA can produce scarless wound healing.
• HA has antioxidant properties.
• HA detoxifies the body.
• HA provides form and shape to the body.

See startling photos that document for the first time the age-reversal properties of this natural molecule.

Number of Pages: 240
ISBN#: 0-9705640-6-6
Price: $19.95
Books can be purchased through Here and Now Books:
www.hereandnowbooks.com
Phone: 909-599-0840
Fax: 909-599-0430

< 196 >

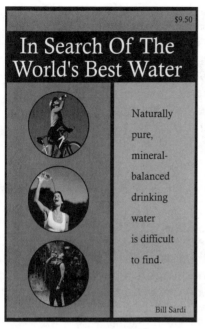

In Search Of The
World's Best Water

$9.50

Naturally

pure,

mineral-

balanced

drinking

water

is difficult

to find.

Bill Sardi

Water, water, everywhere, but so little to drink. So true, for less than 1 percent of the world's water supply is fit to drink. Most is salt water, some is locked up in glaciers, and much of the remainder is either contaminated or unpalatable. It's been said that 80 percent of the world's diseases emanate from impure water. In the western world, human populations have been lulled into the idea that tap water, which is generally safe, is also ideal for health. While tap water is disinfected with chlorine, thus preventing water-borne diseases such as typhoid and dysentery, scientists now admit that by-products of chlorine are a likely cause of cancer (kidneys, bladder, brain, stomach).

Home water filters remedy this problem but don't overcome mineral imbalances. Distilled water is tasteless and dilutes mineral concentrations. Municipal water is softened so it will work in your clothes and dish washer, and so you can bathe without a mineral scum on your body. But softened water is loaded with sodium, which isn't ideal for health. For decades researchers have known that sudden-death heart attack is linked to a lack of magnesium in drinking water. With this in mind, this author went in search of an ideal drinking water, one that is rich in magnesium, calcium balanced, and low in sodium. The worldwide search narrowed down to a handful of bottled waters.

Number of Pages: 208
ISBN#: 0-9705640-9-0
Price: $9.50
Books can be purchased through Here and Now Books:
www.hereandnowbooks.com
Phone: 909-599-0840
Fax: 909-599-0430

< 197 >

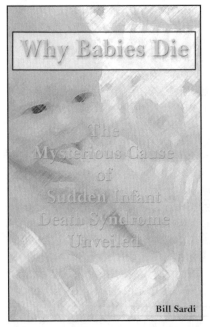

Why Babies Die

The Mysterious Cause of Sudden Infant Death Syndrome Unveiled

Bill Sardi

Did they know about the cause of sudden infant death during Bible times? Whatever does cause unexplainable death among babies has till now eluded detection. For a time, modern medicine was distracted by the use of infant monitors which reduced the risk of SIDS.

What common factor explains why babies....

• Reduce their risk of SIDS by sleeping on their backs
• Increase their risk of SIDS during winter months
• Increase their risk of SIDS with birth order
• Increase their risk of SIDS with infection or fever
• Increase their risk of SIDS with the age of the baby mattress
• Increase their risk of SIDS at infant care centers

The SIDS factor is invisible, non-odorous, transient, and extremely deadly. Now you can learn about the real cause of SIDS.

Number of Pages: 80
ISBN#: 0-9705640-2-3
Price: $7.00
Books can be purchased through Here and Now Books:
www.hereandnowbooks.com
Phone: 909-599-0840
Fax: 909-599-0430

< 198 >

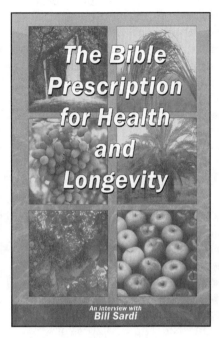

The Bible Prescription for Health and Longevity

An interview with
Bill Sardi

Learn how "God's chosen people" achieved a 70-year life span 3000 years before modern man.

Learn how God made it possible for Adam and Noah to live for hundreds of years.

Learn why the fruits and vegetables provided to the "lost tribe of Israel" delivered more anti-oxidants (anti-rusting agents) than popularly consumed fruits and vegetables today.

Learn how nature's antibiotics, the "bitter herbs" described in the Bible, may save mankind from coming epidemics.

Learn why people in Israel, both now and in the past, experience very low rates of arthritis and osteoporosis as well as maintain youthful hormone levels, because of an unusual concentration of a mineral in the soil.

Learn how the Biblical laws concerning pure food and clean water helped the Israelites live longer and healthier.

Learn how God's unusual provision of omega-3 oils in flax seed and fish protected the Israelites from disease.

Learn why God prescribed that livestock be "grass fed."

Number of Pages: 80
ISBN#: 0-9705640-7-4
Price: $6.95
Books can be purchased through Here and Now Books:
www.hereandnowbooks.com
Phone: 909-599-0840
Fax: 909-599-0430

< 199 >

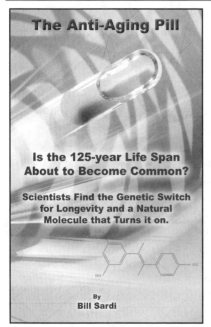

The Anti-Aging Pill

Is the 125-year Life Span About to Become Common?

Scientists Find the Genetic Switch for Longevity and a Natural Molecule that Turns it on.

By
Bill Sardi

Is the 125-year life span about to become common? Scientists find the genetic switch for longevity and a natural molecule that turns it on.

From back cover:
There is a genetic mechanism in all living cells that is far more powerful than any medicine or vitamin that can prolong the life of living cells.

Now scientists discover a small molecule, found in nature, that turns on the longevity switch.

Learn why there is a tremendous upsurge in the number of centenarians around the world, and why millions of people will live beyond the age of 120 years.

Learn why people on two islands, Okinawa and Sardinia, live beyond the age of 100, but for different reasons.

Learn why aging researchers recently began talking about the possibility of an anti-aging pill.

Learn how new discoveries shed light on an environmental phenomenon that has puzzled health researchers for over 70 years.

Learn why Methuselah experienced such unusual longevity.

Learn why the French experience such unusual health and longevity despite a diet rich in fat and calories.

Learn how a pill can now mimic the healthy properties of calorie restriction and red wine consumption.

Number of Pages: 192
ISBN#: 0-9805640-5-8
Price: $19.95
Books can be purchased through Here and Now Books

< 200 >